INSTANT IMAGES

A GUIDE TO USING PHOTOGRAPHY IN THERAPY

Jerry L. Fryrear, Ph.D., A.T.R.
Irene E. Corbit, Ph.D., A.T.R.
Sandra Mason Taylor, MA, LPC, LCDC

KENDALL/HUNT PUBLISHING COMPANY
2460 Kerper Boulevard P.O. Box 539 Dubuque, Iowa 52004-0539

This edition has been printed directly from camera-ready copy.

Copyright © 1992 by Kendall/Hunt Publishing Company

ISBN 0-8403-8182-4

All rights reserved. No part of this publication may be reproduced, stored in a retrieval system, or transmitted, in any form or by any means, electronic, mechanical, photocopying, recording, or otherwise, without the prior written permission of the copyright owner.

Printed in the United States of America.
10 9 8 7 6 5 4 3 2 1

CONTENTS

INTRODUCTION	Page 1
WHY PHOTO ART THERAPY?	Page 3
OVERVIEW OF THIS PROGRAM	Page 7
Supplies	Page 10
The Exercises	Page 12
Outline of Program	Page 15
SECTION ONE: WHO AM I?	Page 19
Assignment # 1: Who Am I in Relation to Nature?	Page 19
Assignment # 2: Who Am I in Relation to Other People?	Page 28
SECTION TWO: WHO AM I REALLY?	Page 36
Assignment # 3: Shadows	Page 36
Assignment # 4: Secrets	Page 48
Assignment # 5: Blind Spots	Page 57
SECTION THREE: WHERE AM I NOW AND WHERE AM I GOING?	Page 64
Assignment # 6: Visual Transitions	Page 64
SECTION FOUR: WHAT IS IN THE WAY?	Page 69
Assignment # 7: Letting Go of Blocks	Page 69
Assignment # 8: Resolving Conflicts	Page 78
SECTION FIVE: WHO ARE WE?	Page 87
Assignment # 9: Defining our Partnership	Page 87
SECTION SIX: WHERE ARE WE NOW AND WHERE ARE WE GOING?	Page 91
Assignment # 10: Visual Transitions as Partners	Page 91
SECTION SEVEN: WHERE HAVE I BEEN THESE PAST FEW WEEKS?	Page 97

i

Assignment # 11: Review and Summary	Page 97
REFERENCES	Page 102
SOME FURTHER READING	Page 104

INSTANT IMAGES

A Guide to Using Photography in Therapy

Jerry L. Fryrear, Irene E. Corbit, and Sandra Mason Taylor

INTRODUCTION

The purpose of this program is to provide a series of guided photographic and artistic exercises that will aid in therapy and personal growth. No special artistic or photographic talent is necessary for either therapist or client, although it is assumed that therapists are knowledgeable about therapy and personality theory. Directions for the assignments are complete within this manual, including lists of supplies, the rationale for each assignment, and instructions on the art work and processing of the work. The instructions are worded for, and directed toward, the client, so that therapists can provide copies of the assignments to clients if they so desire. Because it is necessary when working with cameras for one person to photograph another, the clients are called "partners" throughout, meaning that two people are working together on the camera work and on at least some of the processing, although they may work on the art independently. When working with individuals, the therapist becomes the "partner" and will not carry out the assignments as an equal, but will act as a therapist. When working with groups, we recommend dividing the group into pairs or perhaps triads for the exercises and initial processing of the art work, then recombining the group for a second level processing session.

Therapists who use these activities with their clients will find that they can use the entire program with couples; parts of the program with individuals, excluding the activities examining the relationship between partners; or they can use the program with groups by dividing the group into duos for the assignments, and recombining the entire group for parts of the processing segments. We have found that, in groups, there are usually two levels of processing. The first level, the most intimate and personal, is between the partners. The second level, still meaningful but less intense, takes place when the group members share their experiences with the entire group. We believe that it is important to allow the first level before expecting group members to share with the group as a whole.

Although the manual is presented as a complete program, therapists may elect to use selected assignments to supplement an ongoing therapeutic program of a different nature. If a client is struggling with issues regarding members of the opposite sex, for example, the therapist may wish to use the assignments having to do with one's relationship with other people.

WHY PHOTO ART THERAPY?

Why photo art therapy? We have found, through more than ten years of developing these techniques, that the combination of photographs and art work is a powerful tool for enabling and facilitating one in the ever-present challenge of living a more fulfilling life. The photo art therapy activities in this program are primarily visual, many of the activities also add movement, all of the activities include discussion with a therapist, a group or a partner, and the entire program becomes a metaphor for change.

Visual therapies have advantages that are not available with talking therapies. Wadeson (1980) has discussed several of these advantages. First of all, we, as humans, tend to think in images as well as words. Before we learned to speak, we learned to visualize. Further, these early developmental visualizations are deep-rooted within our personalities, and visual techniques of therapy allow access to early emotions and visual memories more readily than does talking. A recent participant in this photo art therapy program put it this way: "Words can be manipulated and can obscure the truth, but art, in its many forms, bypasses words and darts straight to the soul. It works out things that words often would not know how to explain."

Wadeson writes that imagery is a primary component of unconscious phenomena such as dreams, daydreams, and fantasies. Visual therapies, using art and photographs, allow a dream, fantasy, or experience to be depicted without a laborious and incomplete translation into words. Some experiences simply cannot be described, but they can be drawn or depicted.

Wadeson also reminds us that the art object itself has permanence, and can be considered and addressed as an object outside of the self. This objectification of internal emotions, fantasies, conflicts, frustrations, and so forth is very helpful in making concrete and tangible internal events that are difficult to acknowledge and confront. A participant in our program reported: "The photos themselves were very revealing, especially in being able to see your body language. In one picture of myself the facial expression and body language brought tears. I could visibly see my own loneliness and pain. I knew it was there, but the photo made it so profound. I knew I could not deny this loneliness any longer."

Because the art object is more or less permanent, it provides a record of change, not subject to the distortions of human memory. People can see patterns, emerging themes, and relationships among the assignments that may have not been clear earlier. One woman who worked through the photo art therapy program had this to say: "Some of the photographs were amazing! Photographs are a unique way to deal with emotional and therapeutic issues because of their ability to capture a moment entirely and exactly the way it is. The truth in that time frame of the photo can be referred to again and again and that is a valuable tool--the images remain constant."

This photo art therapy program is structured, to be sure, but not so structured that there is no room for creativity on the part of participants. To the contrary, the creative-expressive nature of the activities is one of the most therapeutic qualities of the program. Creativity and artistic expression is energizing and enlivening. The enlivening and freeing nature of the photo art therapy program was described by a client in the following way: "The use of the visual art materials along with the photos enabled me to first privately process my subconscious thoughts in a free and spontaneous manner. Then with my partner, verbal processing and discussion seemed so natural." In this program there is ample room for individual creativity within the structure.

Another advantage of this photo art therapy program is its multimodal nature. As McNiff has stated (1987, p. 261), "...the psyche expresses itself in a variety of forms. Individual expressive styles differ, and more than one expressive modality may be useful." By providing a multimodal program, we allow the individual to experience multiple avenues for change and personal growth. One client may respond most to photographs, another to the drawings, still another to the movement. All clients seem to benefit from the verbal sharing part of the program.

We believe that the "metaphor for change" aspect of the photo art therapy program is important and significant. As we all know, therapeutic change is extremely difficult. Furthermore, personal growth programs are only successful if, sooner or later, a client makes some changes in his or her life. Many of the activities in this program provide for metaphorical change within the activity. Change is illustrated metaphorically by different poses, different photographs depicting those poses, drawings, collages, and other artistic media. A participant stated it well: "I knew where I was and where I wanted to be, but I was having much difficulty taking actions on the decisions that I knew I had to make. By symbolizing the steps I needed to take, it became more clear and I felt the decisions to be right. I was unable to take these steps before. Now I am taking them and they are not as difficult as I had imagined. Taking the photograph, arranging it, and physically drawing in symbolic terms creates a way to mentally accomplish your goals."

OVERVIEW OF THIS PROGRAM

For those of you who are planning to use the manual as a complete program, we encourage you to follow the assignments as they are presented. The manual follows a logical progression and the later assignments build on earlier ones.

Because of the nature of the photo art therapy assignments, it will be necessary for clients to work with someone else throughout the project. The assignments are designed for partners who will assist each other. It is important that the partners are willing to stick together for the duration of the project (about 16 weeks) and that they are willing to help each other with personal and perhaps emotional issues.

More than two people can work together. It may happen that there are an odd number of people in a group. Simply translate the instructions for partners to instructions for trios, and the three people can carry out the assignments in the same manner as two. Allow one third more time for the assignments.

At the beginning of each assignment in the program, we provide a short rationale for the assignment, that will elaborate on the basic points just outlined. We think you will see that each assignment has its particular reason for being, and that, if carried out in the spirit presented, can be very helpful in therapy and personal growth.

We do want to add one note of caution. Ask your clients to take care of themselves in groups or pairs. They should share personal, intimate information only to the extent that they feel secure about confiding that information. Otherwise, save that information to entrust with the therapist or someone with whom they can be completely trusting. A partner or group member may be trustworthy, but may not appreciate the intimate nature of some revelations. For example, if one confides to one's partner that one was molested as a child, one needs to know that the partner will treat that information confidentially and discreetly. If your clients are working as partners in a group, then the issue of confidentiality is even more pressing.

The subject of confidentiality is an important issue that needs to be addressed at the beginning of any project such as this. Partners and/or group members must acknowledge the fact that to accomplish growth work, a certain amount of personal vulnerability is inevitable. Partners will be well advised to agree to treat each other's statements with respect and privacy. Nonetheless, with all best intentions, partners and/or group members are only human and sometimes personal information is imprudently repeated.

Another important issue to consider is the prospect that some forgotten memories of traumatic events may surface during the art work. Art is a medium that is known to elicit repressed or suppressed information, and it is possible that clients may experience strong emotions during one or more of the assignments. Therapists must be personally and professionally prepared to handle strong emotions on the part of clients.

One other caution: Some hospitals forbid cameras on their units, and have a set policy against photographing patients. Therapists must clarify with the hospital administration that the photographs and the art work would be the property of the individual patient, and that patients' work would involve only their own photographs and would not include photographs of other patients. One art therapy intern used photo art therapy on a hospital adolescent ward, unaware that hospital policy forbids photographs. She had the unpleasant duty of requiring that the adolescents return their photo art therapy posters. Had she discussed the nature of the therapy sessions with the unit supervisor before she began, it is possible that she would have had permission to carry out the project.

Supplies

Here is what you need:

1. A Polaroid 600 camera.

2. Enough film for at least 35 snapshots for each client. Polaroid 600 film is packaged 10 exposures/pack.

3. Art materials. The following are recommended:

    Eight or ten sheets of white poster board per person. You can buy 24" X 28" sheets and cut them in two.

    One box of colored marking pens per person.

    One box of Cray pas oil pastels or crayons per person.

    One package of assorted colors tissue paper per person.

    One package of assorted colors construction paper per person.

    Five sheets of drawing paper, 12" x 18", per person.

    One 9" square box per person. Boxes are available at packaging stores, or you can make your own. It should have a top. If 9" boxes are not available, use ones that are slightly smaller or larger. Even shoe boxes will work, but of course, they will not be uniform cubes.

Several glue sticks, or bottles of paper paste. We do not recommend that you use liquid glue because it causes colors from construction paper and tissue paper to bleed through the photographs.

Several pairs of scissors.

Assorted colors small ribbons and yarn.

Several old magazines with lots of pictures.

Notebook paper and pencils.

You may also want to get colored feathers, spangles, glitter, puff paints, and anything else you might have at home or see in a crafts store. As you progress through the exercises, you will probably think of other supplies that would enhance your clients' creations. Don't hesitate to use anything that strikes your fancy.

The Exercises

The photo art therapy exercises we have designed for this self-directed project are described and explained one at a time. We suggest you follow the sequence as it is presented, and go through one assignment at a time, approximately one per week. Ideally, you will need to schedule two or three hours of uninterrupted time to devote to the program, but time constraints being what they are, you may have to get by with an hour and a half for groups and an hour for individuals. After each assignment, clients will find it helpful to display their art work where they will see it often, as a reminder and a cue for understanding and integration of the new material. There are eleven assignments in all. As we describe the assignments, we will sometimes use "he" or "him" and sometimes "she" or "her" in order to avoid the awkward "he/she" option. We hope you won't find that too confusing.

We begin with assignments that will help clients to understand who they are in relation to nature and to other people. Following these first two assignments, we ask them to take a closer and more penetrating look at themselves, depicting and discussing the "dark side" of the personality, and divulging secrets. A reminder: Clients should divulge only those secrets that they feel trusting enough to share. Encourage your clients to protect themselves, particularly in groups.

On the other side of the spectrum, it is easy to be modest and not admit strengths and positive qualities. Other people can see our good qualities easier than we can, so the next assignment asks partners to point out good qualities to each other, so that they can then pose for photos that symbolize those qualities.

After the first several assignments, clients will understand themselves better than they ever have. Using this new understanding, we ask, "Where are you now in your life, and where are you going?" We call this assignment "visual transitions." Transitions, we understand, are not smooth or easy. There are frustrating blocks to overcome and conflicts that rob us of our energy. The next assignments address these two issues, blocks and conflicts, with an eye toward letting go of blocks and resolving internal conflicts.

At this point in the program, clients have taken a long and interesting look at themselves and have helped each other in the process. Now we turn to the partnership, the relationship. This particular exercise is most relevant for partners who live together or otherwise associate outside of the therapy sessions, but can be used with the partners in a group because by now they know each other very well. Who are they as a couple, where are they now in the relationship, and where are they going?

The final assignment of the program is designed to help

clients "sum up" the entire experience and to put it into perspective.

Following each of the assignments, we offer two examples. Sandra and Evie, friends and business partners, graciously agreed to complete all of the assignments together and to allow us to print photographs of their art work and their remarks about the work and about the assignments. These examples are not meant to show you or your clients how to do the assignments, but to give you an idea of how two partners went about it. Your clients' art work may be much different.

Finally, if you want to do some reading on art therapy and photography, we list a few books that represent the core literature in the field.

Outline of Program

1. Who Am I?

    A. Who am I in relation to nature?
    1. Brief explanation.
    2. Supplies needed.
    3. Photo Art Therapy Assignment # 1: Who Am I in relation to:

        The earth.

        The sky.

        The water.

        The animals.

        The plants.
    4. Processing the assignment with your partner.
    5. Evie and Sandra.

    B. Who am I in relation to other people?
    1. Brief explanation.
    2. Supplies needed.
    3. Photo Art Therapy Assignment # 2: Who am I in relation to:

        Women.

        Men.

        Children.
    4. Processing the assignment with your partner.
    5. Evie and Sandra.

2. Who Am I, Really?

    A. Shadows

        1. Brief discussion of the "shadow" parts of one's personality.

        2. Supplies needed.

        3. Photo Art Therapy Assignment # 3: Depicting the positive and negative dimensions of the dark side.

        4. Processing the assignment with your partner.

        5. Evie and Sandra.

    B. Secrets

        1. Brief explanation.

        2. Supplies needed.

        3. Photo Art Therapy Assignment # 4: Depicting the secret facets of one's personality.

        4. Processing the assignment with your partner.

        5. Evie and Sandra.

    C. Blind Spots

        1. Brief explanation.

        2. Supplies needed.

        3. Photo Art Therapy Assignment # 5: Seeing your blind spots, recognizing your strengths.

        4. Processing the assignment with your partner.

        5. Evie and Sandra.

3. Where Am I Now And Where Am I Going?

A. Brief explanation.

B. Supplies needed.

C. Photo Art Therapy Assignment # 6: Visual transitions.

D. Processing the assignment with your partner.

E. Evie and Sandra.

4. What Is In The Way?

   A. Letting Go of Blocks.

      1. Brief discussion.

      2. Supplies needed.

      3. Photo Art Therapy Assignment # 7: Depicting and letting go of blocks.

      4. Processing the assignment with your partner.

      5. Evie and Sandra.

   B. Resolving Conflicts.

      1. Brief explanation.

      2. Supplies needed.

      3. Photo Art Therapy Assignment # 8: Depicting and resolving conflicts.

      4. Processing the assignment with your partner.

      5. Evie and Sandra.

5. Who Are We?

   A. Brief explanation.

   B. Supplies needed.

   C. Photo Art Therapy Assignment # 9: Defining our partnership.

D. Processing the assignment.

E. Evie and Sandra.

6. Where Are We Now, And Where Are We Going?

A. Brief explanation.

B. Supplies needed.

C. Photo Art Therapy Assignment # 10: Visual transitions as partners.

D. Processing the assignment.

E. Evie and Sandra.

7. Where Have I Been These Past Few Weeks?

A. Brief explanation.

B. Supplies needed.

C. Photo Art Therapy Assignment # 11: A review and summary of the program.

D. Processing and summarizing the project.

E. Evie and Sandra.

8. For Those of You Who Want to Know More, Some Further Reading.

SECTION ONE: WHO AM I?

Assignment # 1. Who Am I In Relation To Nature?

Brief Explanation

We are inextricably bound to nature, and part of it. Unfortunately, in our technological world we have lost track of many of the rhythms and relationships that exist between people and nature. That is especially true for those of us who live in the city. We have forgotten that all of nature is interrelated and interdependent and that we are very much a part of nature. The purpose of this first assignment is to help you regain that sense of being a part of nature.

Andreas Feininger, through words and photographs, has presented eloquent testimony to the beauties and mysteries of nature and our confused and contradictory, often foolhardy dealings with the natural world (1956, 1977, 1983, 1986). In one of his early photographic works on nature, Feininger wrote:

"Walk on a dew-fresh morning in the forest and attune yourself to your environment until you feel part of it. You will find wonders in the diversity of life, the intricacy of its manifestations. Wherever you look, there is life. A dormant seed, small as a grain of sand, bears within its tiny shell the future flowering plant. A squirrel watches from its perch, half-hidden behind the trunk of a tree. A deermouse scurries in the underbrush. A spider waits patiently in its web. Armies of caterpillars chew away the leaves. Each life depends upon another, pursuing or pursued in the great battle for survival, the vanquished furnishing the victor with a meal. Worms tunnel the ground converting leaf mold to humus. Fungi and bacteria break down decaying matter into organic compounds which in time will nourish new life.

The air itself vibrates with sound and motion, the wingbeats of insects, the song and call of birds, the ceaseless whispering of boughs and leaves rustled by the gentle morning winds.

You become aware of the interdependence of all life, animals and plants, all of nature's creations, each dependent upon others for sustenance or protection. And you realize with sharp clarity that you, too, are part of this immensity of nature, a humble yet important part, earth-bound, mortal, dependent for survival upon animal and plant, and that the molecules and atoms that constitute your body are identical with those that compose the rocks, the plants, the animals, the earth, moon, sun, and stars."(1956, p.17).

Supplies Needed

1. Camera
2. Film for five exposures each.

3. One sheet of poster board each.
4. Assorted art supplies, scissors, and glue.

Assignment

Think of yourself in relation to the natural elements of earth, sky, water, animals, and plants, and imagine how you would pose to depict those five relationships. Talk it over with your partner. The poses can be literal or metaphorical. When you have decided on the poses, have your partner take the snapshots. You will probably want to go outdoors for these photos.

Don't worry too much about composing the perfect photograph, with the exact background you want. Because you will be adding other artistic media, you can draw in mountains, the seashore, birds, trees, other people, anything you want. You can also find photographs in magazines that you can add to your composition.

Now that you and your partner have five snapshots each, think about how you would compose the five photographs on a piece of poster board to create a self-portrait in relation to nature. You may want to cut out the photographic images from their frames before gluing them to the poster board, and to add to the background of the poster board using the other art supplies, such as the marking pens, tissue paper, oil pastels, and construction paper. Hint: When you cut out images from the polaroid prints, peel off the backing before gluing the image. Otherwise, the back will come off in the future and the image will fall off the poster board. There will be a faint image of the photograph on the inside of the backing. Some people have incorporated that faint image into their art work, as you may wish to do.

Caution: The Polaroid Corporation advises against cutting apart the photographs because the developing chemicals within the layers of the photograph are mildly irritating to the skin. In ten years of working with the photographs in this way, we have not had any problems, but we advise you to wash your hands after handling any pictures that have been cut apart, and to avoid rubbing the eyes. When working with children or people who may be mentally handicapped, we advise the therapist do the cutting.

You and your partner will each complete a poster board portrait using the photos and art supplies. As you prepare your portrait board, try to adopt a playful and excited attitude. There is no right or wrong way to do the art work. Don't worry about whether the final work is artistic or not. The process is important, not the product. Trust your impulses and your innate creativity, and let your unconscious be your guide. You will find that, if you play with the materials, move them around on the poster board, try different colors and shapes, that a natural process will emerge. Some colors, shapes and relationships feel "right" for you. Go with that. Don't worry about what anyone else might think.

Processing

In this and all future assignment processing, adopt a listening and supporting attitude with your partner. Here are some DOs and DON'Ts:

DO listen carefully, without arguing.

DO encourage your partner.

DO try to understand your partner.

DO share your own experiences.

DON'T criticize.

DON'T analyze your partner's creations. It is all right to analyze your own, just don't get too carried away.

DON'T make fun of or belittle your partner's efforts, or your own efforts. Treat the work with respect.

Show your portrait board to your partner and describe and explain it. Listen to your partner's narration about his or her portrait board. Avoid trying to analyze your portraits or the portraits of your partner, that is, pronouncing what the photographs "mean." Instead of analyzing, help your partner to understand and learn by encouraging, pointing out consistencies, and sharing your own experiences.

During the processing period, you may find that you want to change your portrait board. You may want to add or subtract photos, change colors and forms, or otherwise tinker with it. Fine, go ahead. That is part of learning about yourself. Talk about the changes with your partner.

Take as long as you want with the art work and the processing, and then give yourself a few days off before starting the next assignment. It is always good to allow new information and new understanding to "incubate" for a few days before adding more.

Evie and Sandra

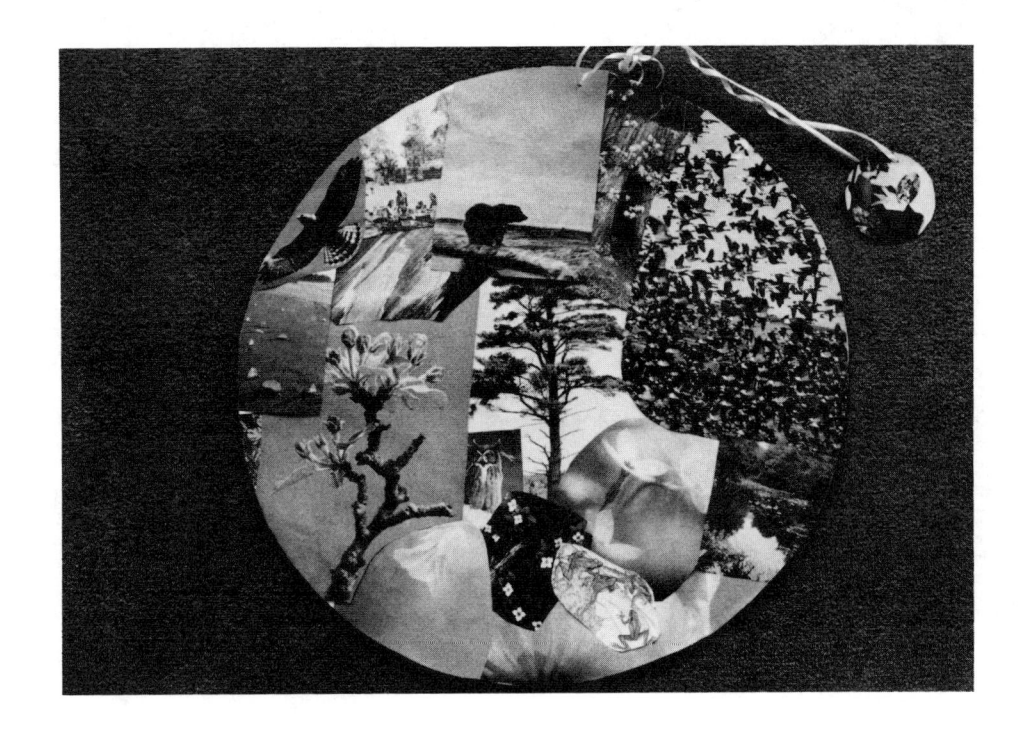

Evie: "The assignment is to look at myself in relation to nature. At this point in life I am longing to be more in touch with nature. With everything from the flowers in my backyard to the forays I used to take to see geese come in to South Texas. I want to go to Alaska. I want to go out walking and be in touch with things that are natural. That's a really rich part of life for me. Instead I find myself at this juncture starting a new business, starting a Ph.D. program, locked in at my computer.

This is a different kind of creativity, but doing this project made me realize how much I miss being connected, so I put myself in a different circle, not really attached to the mandala of nature for me. I'm swinging unattached, swinging through the air, and missing the attachment."

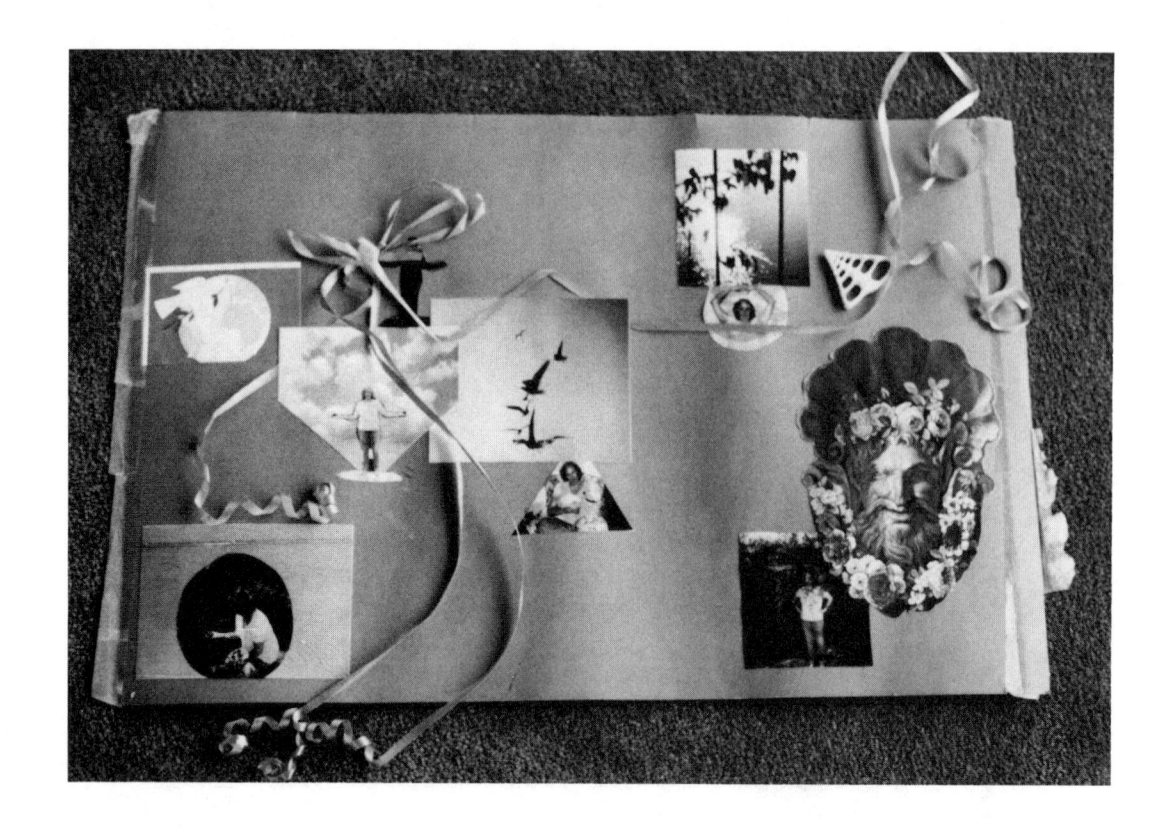

Sandra: "As I was doing this poster, the first thing I started looking for were pictures of the sky. I put myself in the sky because of my longing to be off the ground. I flew airplanes when I was young and loved it. I am thinking after doing this poster that I will go back and pick flying up again. That was really important to me and a source of great contentment.

My connection with animals right now is very limited because I live in a small town house. I have a small triangular picture of me with my teddy bear. I also have birds, because I love to watch them and that's also another connection to the sky.

As far as my connection to the water, I feel whole and complete when I am around water. I live in a town house complex that has a small lake. I go and sit sometimes and just look at it and feel rested. It's a really important element in my life.

The plants and flowers I have limited contact with right now. They have always been important to me. I need fresh flowers and have them around me all the time in my office and at home too.

I have the pictures connected with a ribbon because it seems to me that they are all necessary to my life, they are all connected, and as I like it to be light and playful I used bright colored ribbons."

Assignment # 2: Who Am I In Relation To Other People?

Brief Explanation

We interact with other people every day, but rarely do we examine and try to understand our orientation toward others. In this assignment, you are asked to examine your relationship to women, to men, and to children, to people in general, not to a specific woman, a certain man, a particular child. A better understanding of your relationship to others will help you to understand your basic orientation toward a relationship at its beginning, as well as help to explain why you act in certain ways around people you know just because they are a certain gender or age.

Supplies Needed

1. Camera
2. Film for three exposures each.
3. At least one sheet of poster board each.
4. Assorted art supplies, scissors, and glue.

Assignment

Think of yourself and your basic stance, or orientation, toward women, men, and children. Imagine how you would pose to show these three relationships. Talk it over with your partner.

If you are stuck, and can't think how to carry out this assignment, here is one idea that may help. The psychologist William Schutz (1958) suggested that there are three major orientations we have toward other people. The three are Inclusion, Control, and Affection. Furthermore, we both desire inclusion, control and affection from others, and we express inclusion, control and affection toward others. In carrying out this assignment, think about how much you desire to be included in children's activities, in men's activities, in women's activities. How much do you include them in your activities? How much do you want to control others? How much control and direction do you want from them? Do you express affection toward children? Toward men? Toward women? Or does that make you uncomfortable and embarrassed? How much affection do you want other people to display toward you? Do you like to be hugged? Kissed?

Let your partner help you decide on your three poses. When you are ready, have your partner take your three photographs depicting the relationships. Now trade off and take your partner's photographs.

You and your partner now have three photos each. Compose the photos on the piece of poster board in whatever manner you choose to show yourself in your orientation toward those three groups of people; women, men and children. Use the other art materials, and perhaps pictures from magazines to embellish the art work. Many people prefer to cut out the images from the background of the Polaroid frame before gluing them down on the board. In our experience, some people feel too restricted with only one piece of poster board for all three relationships. If you want to use a separate sheet of poster board for each of the three, go ahead.

Processing

The processing, or sharing phase of this assignment is somewhat more ticklish than the preceding one because your partner is a member of one of the three groups of people. If your partner is a man, then your explanation and discussion of your relationship toward men will encompass your partnership. He may take whatever you say personally. Likewise, you are a member of one of the classes of people to which he will refer. Be open and encouraging of each other, without taking a defensive stance. The processing will be most helpful if the two of you see it as a time to share rather than to attack or analyze. Listen, be supportive, try to understand, share your own experiences and feelings. If you do not understand what your partner is trying to say, put it in your own words and repeat it back. Take as much time as necessary.

While you are thinking about and talking about your composition, pay attention to what is _not_ there. For example, are there any elderly people in your composition? When you thought about children, what ages came to mind? Did you think of adolescents, or infants? If you want, you can use the structure of this assignment to explore your relationships with more specific groups of people--the elderly, adolescents, babies, coworkers, neighbors, in-laws. Simply substitute for men, women and children the question, "Who am I in relation to co-workers?" (for example) and repeat the assignment.

As with the first assignment, if you want to modify your composition, by all means do so! As you gain understanding of yourself, you may see relationships more clearly and want to depict them differently. Talk it over with your partner.

Take a few days off before beginning assignment # 3. Put your compositions from the first two assignments where you can see them every day. Don't be surprised if you gain insights when you are not directly working on the program. Maybe even in your dreams.

Evie and Sandra

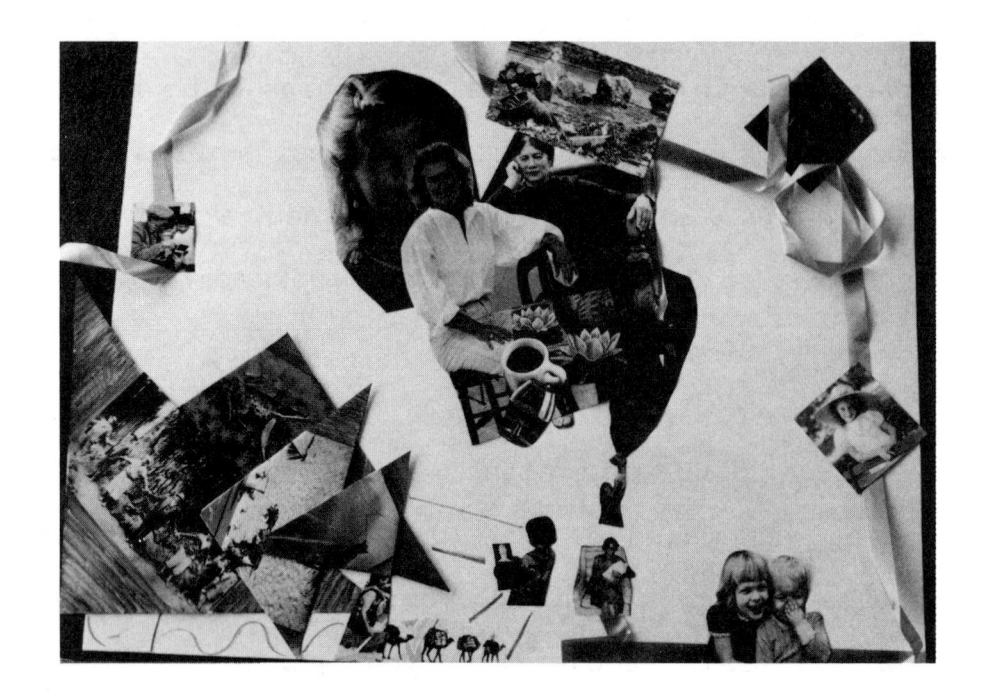

Evie: "Who am I in relation to other people? Central to my poster is my relationship to women--that seems the richest part of my life right now. My life is full of interesting, competent, exciting, strong women and they are in the forefront of the picture. That is where the passion is. There is a picture of me holding the fire out of which come both relaxation (coffee and brandy) and nature (the water lilies and women of different ages and different attitudes). There is a young woman, a child-woman, and an older woman. The remarkable thing about this is that after cutting out the very central photograph from a magazine, a friend saw it and said, "Oh, I know this woman. Would you like to meet her?" And that very week I met her. She is a fascinating playwright and somebody I would like to know.

The relationship to children is part of my past at the moment.

I really miss having small children. I miss watching them grow up. I miss that part.

My relationship to men is off to the left side, the unconscious side of my poster. They are in triangles because my relationships right now with several of the important men in my life are sharp around the edges. They are not flowing easily and smoothly. They have jagged edges. There is a frog in this picture because I believe that you have to kiss a lot of frogs before you find a prince. I found that to be true in my life with men.

Also there, in a very real way, is a collage of crossing the desert on camels, rafting, and some of the fun things I do with my husband. He is not really in the picture right now; he is halfway around the world so that accounts for the placement of men in the picture. I don't know the environment here in Houston well enough to establish those relationships and keep them the way they need to be with him gone, so I am reluctant to do anything but put it on hold."

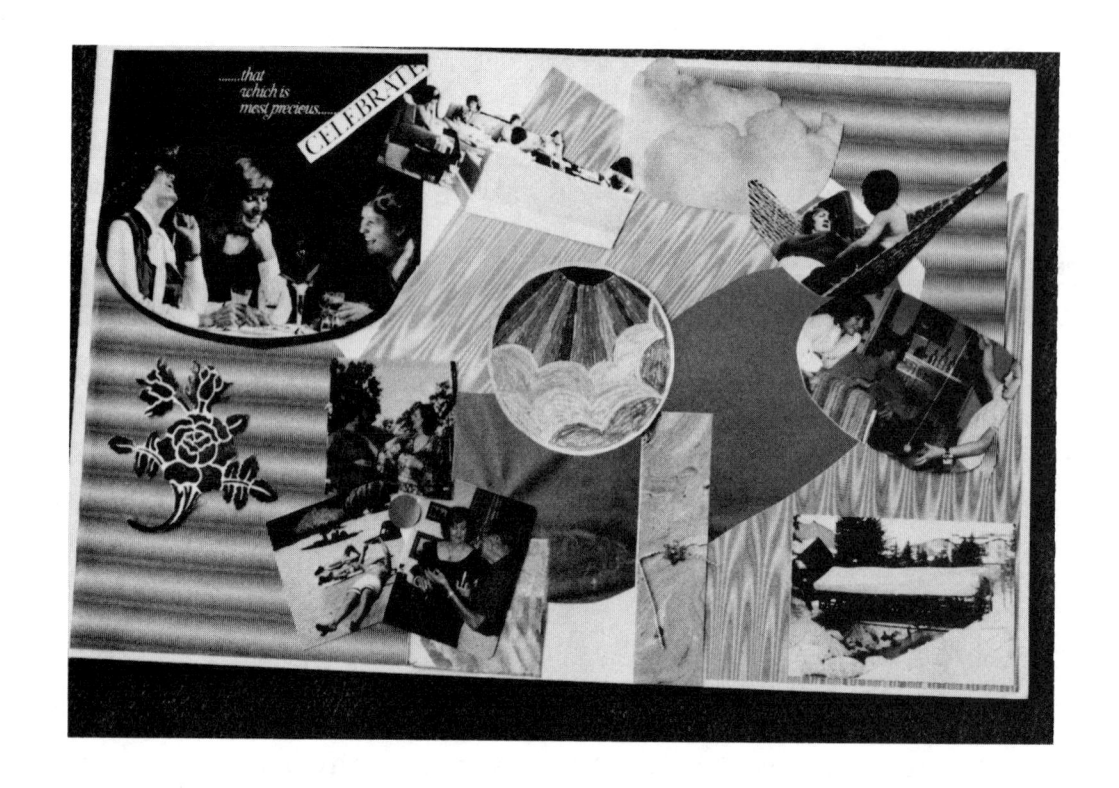

Sandra: "In the center of my picture I have a mandala that I drew some time ago that means relationship for me. The sun breaking through stormy clouds is the way a lot of my relationships have become. I have more women than men in my life right now. I celebrate with them. I consider these relationships precious. The men that I work with are mostly younger than I am, we have a mutual teaching of each other as I have shown by one of the pictures with our hands on each other's shoulders. With older men, I have a stance of listening and "being with" although that sometimes is difficult for me.

The children I am around mostly are my grandchildren who of course are very special. I spend a lot of time visiting with my grandsons and celebrating with them doing family things.

I have a covered bridge in this picture which is for me a

pathway to something I don't know about yet in relationships. Probably this signifies new men in my life and it is covered and it is cold and I don't know where that's going to go."

SECTION TWO: WHO AM I, REALLY?

Assignment # 3: Shadows

Brief Explanation

The "shadow" parts of your personality pop up when you least expect it and tend to disrupt and sabotage your attempts at happiness and satisfaction. You usually know when your "shadow" has been operating, after the fact. You say to yourself, "Now, why did I do that?" "That's not like me!" "I wasn't myself last night." Or you catch yourself in the middle of some act or statement, and you want to stop but for some reason are compelled to continue. If you intensely dislike someone you barely know, particularly if it is someone of the same sex, perhaps you are seeing "shadow" qualities of yourself in that other person, and the unconscious recognition of those qualities in yourself leads to the distasteful reaction. James Hall (1990) has defined the shadow succinctly as "That part of your personality that you don't think you have, but suspect you do, and if you do, you hope nobody notices!"

The shadow can take many forms and is present in all of us, in both conscious and unconscious shapes. There are several shadow qualities that are immediately recognizable by most everybody. These are:

<u>The hypocrite.</u> The person who says one thing and does another. Perhaps you have done that yourself.

<u>The pedant</u>, or "know it all." The person who has to straighten out other people by quoting the facts.

<u>The gossip.</u> The person who glories in other people's foibles.

<u>The glutton.</u> Eating and drinking without moderation.

<u>The seductress or seducer.</u> The person who feels compelled to relate to the opposite gender in sexual ways only.

<u>The rescuer or hero</u>. Some people rush in to rescue others when they don't want or need to be helped. Most of us do that from time to time.

<u>The victim or naive child.</u> Some other people always seem to put themselves into predicaments where they really do need to be rescued. They run out of gas on the freeway. They walk in dangerous neighborhoods alone. They pick up strangers.

<u>The passive-helpless person.</u> The person who appears to be helpless but who in fact is not. He or she will wait for others to make decisions, to take charge, to discharge duties. Passive-helpless people never have change for tips, they can't find their

keys, they are always late for appointments.

<u>The miser, or Scrooge.</u> Charles Dickens' character Ebeneezer Scrooge has become almost synonymous with miserliness. As we all know from <u>A Christmas Carol</u> Scrooge was a bitter, unhappy man, driven to hoard his money, obsessed with accumulating wealth without enjoying it. Many of us are unreasonably tight with our resources, accumulating and hoarding selfishly beyond all need to do so for our own security.

<u>The aggressor or warrior</u>. The person who relates to other people with violence or anger. A more subtle variant of the aggressor is the quality of passive aggression. That is, someone who stands by and does not prevent injury or violence when it could be prevented. For instance, you notice that a woman is about to slip on an icy sidewalk and you do not warn her.

You probably were able to recognize some of your acquaintances from these brief descriptions. Less likely is the possibility that you were able to recognize, or at least admit, the shadow qualities in yourself. This assignment asks you to do just that. Think about and admit at least one "shadow" facet of your personality that you would be willing to investigate more thoroughly, in order to accept and then to integrate that quality into your personality in ways that will be to your advantage, rather than to your disadvantage. Such an integration is possible because shadow qualities have both negative and positive attributes. We tend to deny and project onto other people these shadow qualities because we see only the negative side.

Consider the "know it all." Certainly, having knowledge is not an undesirable thing. The trick is "knowing" when to be knowledgeable. One of the authors (JF) was talking with his young niece a few years ago and she remarked, "I wish leaves were money." Whereupon, he "straightened her out" by informing her that, according to the laws of economics, if leaves were money they would still be worthless because of their sheer quantity. The shadowy pedant had popped out unbidden, to spoil the child's fantasy of riches. Not surprisingly, his niece had little else to say the rest of the afternoon, for fear of the consequences. On the other hand, the economics lesson would be perfectly appropriate in an economics class, or if the girl had asked for an explanation.

How about aggression? Anger has its place, and, if used without violence, tells others exactly how we feel without hurting them. Furthermore, aggression is frequently mistaken for assertiveness. Assertiveness is standing up for one's rights without infringing on the rights of others. Aggression does infringe on the rights of others. We often fail to be assertive because we are convinced that, to do so, would be to give in to the aggressor shadow. The recognition and admission of the aggressor shadow allows us to make the distinction between aggression and assertiveness, and to become more assertive while controlling the aggression.

There are other examples. Occasional gluttony is fun. People do sometimes need to be rescued. We can discuss other people without gossiping. In short, every shadow has its positive-negative dimension. The present assignment is designed to help you become more aware of and knowledgeable about one of your "shadows" along its entire dimension from negative to positive. Be assured that you (and all of us) have more than one shadow, but we shall start with just one. You may want to work on others later.

The great psychologist Carl G. Jung wrote, "If we are able to see our own shadow and can bear knowing about it, then a small part of the problem has already been solved."(1968, p. 20).

Supplies Needed

1. Camera.
2. Film for two photographs each.
3. One sheet of poster board each.
4. Assorted art supplies, glue and scissors.

Assignment

During the discussion of the shadow, above, you probably had an inkling of some shadow parts of your own personality. If not, think about times when you have been compelled to do something, or were obsessed with some action or thought. Another hint of the shadow lies in your choices of movies, music, plays and books. What particularly excites you, that you are reluctant to tell your friends about? Remember qualities in other people that you dislike. Perhaps you have those qualities to some extent yourself and don't like to admit it.

We have provided space on pages 46 and 47 to make sketches and notes about your shadow. Use one page and your partner can use the other.

When you have selected one shadow to explore, imagine both ends of a positive-negative dimension related to that shadow quality. Let your partner help with this imagination. When you have the dimension in mind, then explore with your partner how you can depict the two ends of the dimension with poses that can be photographed. Strike the poses and let your partner photograph them. Do the same for your partner.

Mount the two photographs on the poster board in such a way to depict the positive-negative dimension of the shadow quality. Use any art materials you need to augment the depiction.

Processing

Discussing undesirable qualities in ourselves can be embarrassing. By now, however, you and your partner know each other very well and have already admitted to the shadow during the photographic and artistic phases of the assignment. Furthermore, you do not have to show your work to anyone else unless you want to. At this point, simply elaborate on your poster board. Discuss your choice of poses, your use of particular colors and shapes, the relationship of the negative to the positive ends of the shadow dimension. Discuss with your partner how you can convert the negative qualities of the shadow to the positive ones in your everyday life.

As with all assignments in this program, do not attack, belittle, or analyze your partner's efforts. Remember, your partner is trying to be open and honest in an effort at self-understanding. Your partner needs support and a sense of sharing in that difficult enterprise. So do you.

Give yourself a break for about a week. You may want to explore other shadow facets of your personality. Go ahead, but wait for a few days, and make sure that your partner wants to also. If you decide to choose another shadow from your personality to explore, follow the same procedure as outlined above.

Evie and Sandra

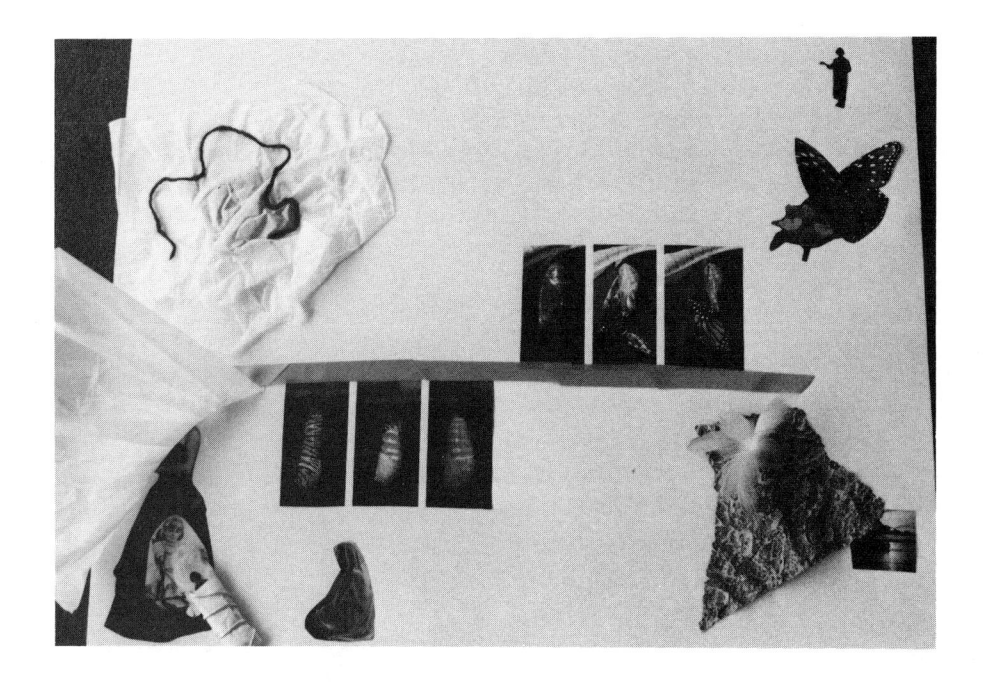

Evie: "The assignment is to explore the shadow parts of myself. What I started with was a covered pile of manure and discovered it is not as covered as I like to think it is. I discovered that it shows through more than I like to admit.

Down on the left hand side, also covered, but you can lift the curtain to see her, is a very elegant southern lady, the way I was brought up and taught to be. I fairly completely dissociated myself from Southern Lady for many years. I took on a profession, a lot of travel, outside involvement, and dropped a southern accent. That is part of shadow for me, a disrespect for the passive way that I was brought up to be.

There is also myself bound in a sort of cocoon. Southern Lady training bound me, in my perception.

Part of this shadow is a Muslim woman. I have lived a lot

among Muslim women and have gained respect for their way of being passive by living with them and understanding them better.

So my cocoon-bound Southern Lady may be evolving. That's the central issue here. Evolving into someone who can be soft, but strong, rubbing the edges off of that passivity. In evolving, able to enjoy the boating theme on the right, the naturalness. I need a return to nature that wouldn't be so constricted. One I wouldn't be so much in rebellion against."

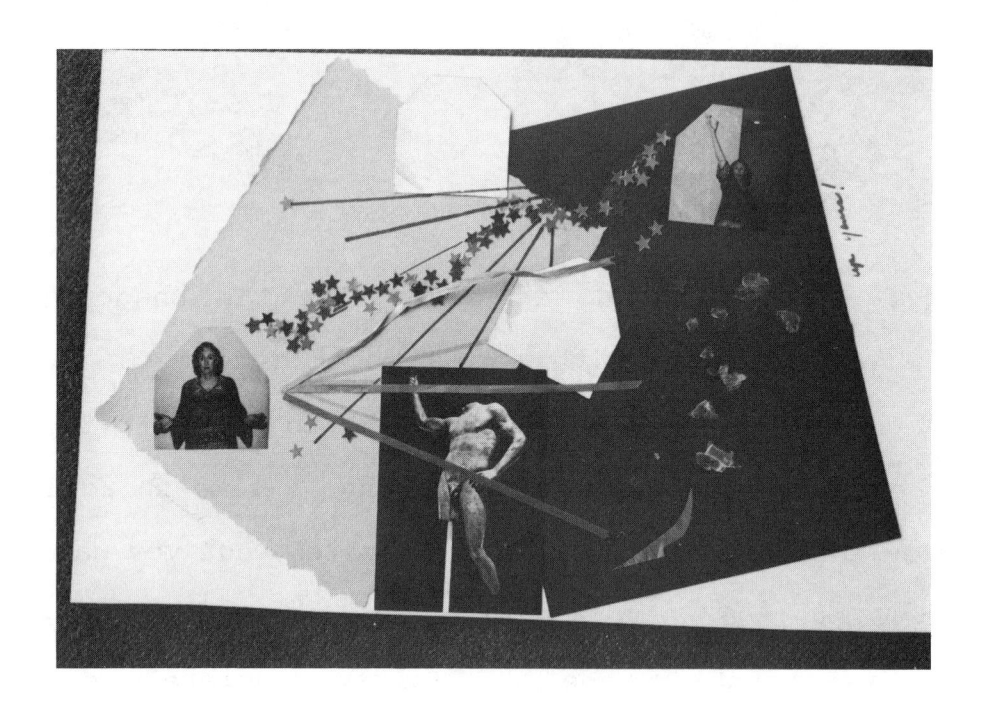

<u>Sandra</u>: "About shadow. It seems to me I spend a lot of my time being reasonable with people and being cool and making sure that everybody gets what they need. Often what I am feeling is wanting to say 'up yours' or something equally rude to people. I think that the people who bring out the shadow side of me are men more than women.

I have some black behind the shadow side and some ladylike

pink behind the other. There is a very strong connection I've shown with the stars in the picture. There is a lot of fallout when I come to the shadow side as I have depicted by the mica that is dripping down from victory."

BLANK PAGE FOR NOTES AND SKETCHES ABOUT MY SHADOW

BLANK PAGE FOR NOTES AND SKETCHES ABOUT MY SHADOW

Assignment # 4: Secrets

Brief Explanation

We all have secrets. The kind of secrets we are discussing here are not secrets about what you have done, but secrets about your personality. Secret ways of thinking about yourself that you have shared with few people, perhaps no one, before.

We are complex, many-faceted humans with a great capacity for sharing and hiding, pretending and admitting, play-acting and being honest. This assignment is designed to help you explore six facets of your personality in more detail than you have up to now. You will find that the previous three assignments will lead naturally into at least one or two of the facets you are about to explore.

One well-organized part of personality is the ability and tendency to play roles. We are different people in different settings. You act one way at work, another way with your family, still another at church. In fact, these are not "merely" roles, but entire complexes of actions, attitudes, expectations, and concepts of self. You have a concept of yourself as a family person, an occupational (or student, or housekeeper) person, a spiritual person, a physical person, a social person, an emotional person. Furthermore, for each of these concepts you display a persona, or a public figure, and for each of the concepts you clasp to yourself a private, or secret figure. You may present to the world a persona of a successful, confident, decisive executive. Underneath, you feel like an imposter and wonder how you get by from day to day without "them" finding out that you are incompetent in your job. Your neighbor is a picture of health and attractiveness. Good figure and a delightful smile. She knows about her abdominal scar and tells no one, yet worries about her "disfigurement."

Carl Jung believed that this other-oriented facade, or persona, must be examined and torn down for true individuality to be possible. We can never become our true selves if we are terribly concerned about our appearance to other people. By exploring our facades, and especially those parts of our personality that we keep secret from other people, we begin to "tear down" the persona in preparation for a more genuine identity.

The purpose of the present assignment is to provide a structure for you to explore and share six different self-concepts, or personas, both public and private. You will complete a "self-portrait box." The six concepts are:
1. physical self,
2. spiritual self,
3. family self,
4. social self,
5. occupational self, and

6. emotional self.

Following this assignment, you may still wish to hide certain parts of your personality in certain settings, but it will be by choice rather than by automatic personal fiat.

The exercise, because it is divided into six parts, will take six different sessions, or one very lengthy one. Some people prefer to approach the box one side at a time, allowing several days between sessions. Other people are uncomfortable with remaining in an unfinished state for several weeks, and prefer to finish the entire box in one setting, or perhaps two. If you find yourself wanting to finish the box, go ahead. Work at your own pace. You and your partner may discover that you are on different schedules for this assignment. If that happens, try to work out a compromise so that you are working together.

Supplies Needed

1. Camera.
2. Film for at least twelve photographs each.
3. One 8" x 8" x 8" (approximate size) cardboard box each.
4. Twelve 8" x 8" squares cut from poster board or drawing paper, each.
5. Assorted art supplies, glue and scissors.
6. A pencil.

Assignment

Lightly, in pencil, label the outside of the boxes with the words Public Physical Self, Public Family Self, Public Social Self, Public Spiritual Self, Public Occupational Self, and Public Emotional Self, one on each side. Label the corresponding insides of the box with Secret Physical Self, Secret Family Self, and so forth opposite the Public labels for each side. When you finish, you should have a cube that is labeled Public Physical Self and, opposite, on the inside, Secret Physical Self on one side, Public Family Self and, opposite, on the inside, Secret Family Self, and so on for the six sides.

With your partner, choose one of the Public sides to begin with. It doesn't matter which one, but you and your partner agree to work on the same concept. Suppose you choose Public Social Self as a starting point. Imagine a pose that would represent your persona as a social being, and have your partner photograph you in that pose. Then, you photograph your partner. Help each other decide on the poses.

Compose your photograph on one of the 8" x 8" squares of paper or cardboard, and augment the photo with your art materials. You may wish to draw in background, attach other pictures from magazines, or whatever would help to depict yourself as a social person.

With your partner helping you, decide how you would depict some secret about yourself and your concept of yourself as a social being. Say, you secretly feel uncomfortable near people of a certain race or culture. This secret will, of course, be something you are willing to share with your partner, but perhaps with no one else. Depict the secret with a pose of your choice and have your partner photograph the pose. Reciprocate.

Compose the secret photograph on another cardboard square and add the other art work. You now have two pieces of art each, your public and secret social selves. Glue the two squares on the appropriately labeled sides of the box. Your public persona will be on the outside and your secret on the inside. When you close the lid, only you know that the secret photograph is inside. From the outside it looks like an ornate photo cube.

Process these first two photographs with each other, sharing and discussing. After you finish with the processing, wait a few days and then choose another side to work on. The entire assignment will take several hours, either in one session or several. When the box is completely finished, you have "put yourself together" in a three-dimensional cube, with both inside and outside dimensions.

Display the photo cube anywhere you want. If you want the secrets inside to be completely private, glue the top of the box closed. Only you and your partner will know that there are also photographs inside. Some people have placed objects inside the box after it was completed to further emphasize the complexity of their personalities.

Processing

Describe and explain your two pieces of art to your partner. Share only as much of the secret as you are comfortable with. Do not pry and coerce if your partner does not want to tell you all.

Evie and Sandra

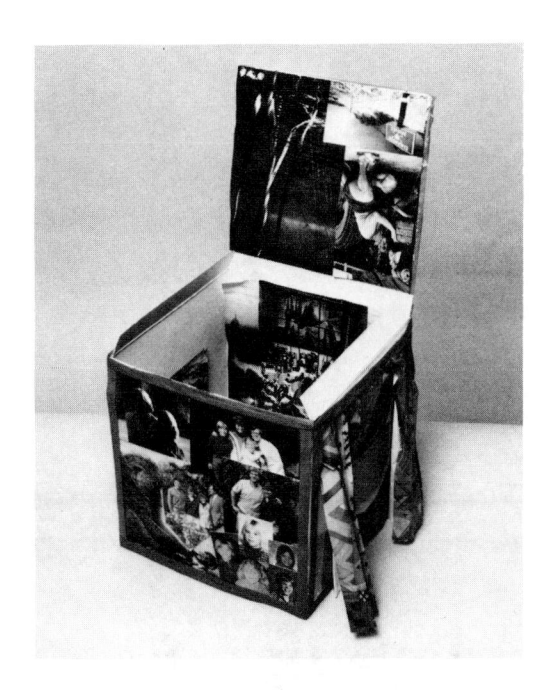

Evie: "The box with six sides that represent the physical, spiritual, family, social, occupational, and emotional self... This was a really fascinating project for me and I found that I wanted to do it all in one sitting. I didn't want to string it out over several weeks because I really got involved in the process and almost couldn't put it aside.

The theme that unites all of the different sides of this on the outside frames is a very extroverted well-adapted social self, and at home. Inside a quieter, introverted self. I know what I need to do to get by in the world and yet the backside of each one of these is a much more retiring side. I came upon the discovery that I probably have not been an extravert all of my life, but an adapted introvert who knows how to do extraversion very well.

As a result, I set aside regular times to both run and meditate after I did this box. I am trying to honor what is real and not have such a drastic split between what I show and what I experience. Very, very interesting project for me."

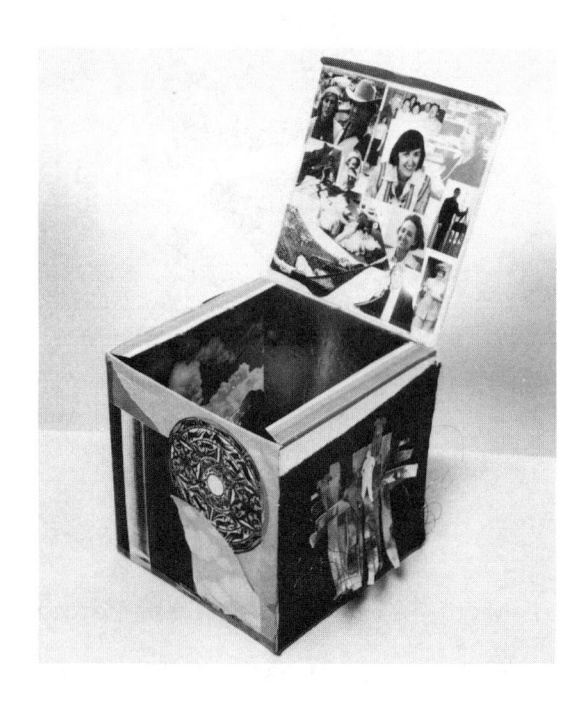

Sandra: "This box was a remarkable experience for me and it

gave me the opportunity to focus on what is happening in my external life right now, and the way I want it to be. I realize that I hide myself more than I thought. That's an old habit left over from the days when I believed it was necessary to protect myself.

On my occupational side, I think that people see me in my everyday life as being busy and strong. I have put a mirror on that side to show how I use Rogerian reflection when I do therapy. I am full of blue sky ideas. The hidden me dreams and works with my hands and loves being alone. The external part of me works at an office and sits at a desk and manages people and does therapy all day long. I long for the time to work with my hands. Because of this exercise, I have gone to Texas Art Supply, bought myself a lot of art supplies, and have set up a room in my house so that I can go in and spend a little time from time-to-time doing creative work. On my occupational side I see my job as being full of excitement and hard work. Some days I feel like I am running up an unending flight of very steep stairs. When it gets too much, I daydream of escaping in my airplane and never coming down. So the inside of my box on by occupational side shows a very small airplane and very big clouds.

My outside spiritual self is interested in <u>The Course of Miracles</u>, zen, and the Tao. I am actively studying these different ways of understanding the world. Inside I am full of wonder and wondering and knowing and not even knowing what it is I know.

My physical self is growing older. I feel some resentment

that I have to spend more time taking care of myself. I'd like to spend my time thinking and not exercising. I have embarked on my new health program because I have realized that this is something that I need to do. I am working on my resentment.

My outside emotional self has visions for the future. It is clear about choices and cheerful about the complexities of life. Inside I still have fantasies of a great love and a life of richness and joy.

I'm not sure about how this exercise has impacted me yet. The experience is still rich in my life. I have the finished box in my living room and as I pick it up and look at it, I think there are a lot of things there for me that I will continue to discover that I need to know about myself."

Assignment # 5:   Blind Spots

Brief Explanation

Lest you are beginning to think all is secrets and shadows, darkness and embarrassments, now we are going to ask you to look at your good qualities. Strangely enough, it is very difficult for people to see their own strengths and positive qualities. Almost from birth, we are taught to be modest, not to brag, to avoid boasting. Think how hard it is to simply say "thank you" to a compliment. We want to deny, to lessen the impact.

Because it is so difficult to see and talk about our good qualities, in this exercise we assign that task to your partner. Your partner will point out your strengths and direct you in the poses that will symbolize those qualities. Your job is to simply accept your partner's direction, and to acknowledge the traits.

Supplies Needed

1. Camera.
2. Film for three photographs each.
3. One piece of poster board each.
4. Assorted art materials, glue and scissors.
5. Two pencils and pages 46-47 of this manual.

Assignment

Turn to pages 60 and 61. Notice that there are spaces for making notes. One of you use page 60 and the other, page 61. Both of you, take a pencil, think about your partner and write down three (or more) qualities that you like and admire about him or her. Opposite each of the qualities, write down an instance when you were aware that your partner had that quality. For example, you remember when she showed she was honest when she received too much change at the supermarket and returned it.

Direct your partner in the kinds of poses that you think would represent each of those three qualities in him or her, and take the snapshots. When your partner is directing you, do not argue or try to demean or belittle the statements or poses. If necessary, pretend that you are an actor and are being directed to play a role.

Collect the three photographs of yourself and the page of notes written about you by your partner. Using the photos and the notes, construct a self-portrait board on the poster board, augmenting the photos with the other art materials. This is no time to be modest.

Processing

This next part is hard, but do it anyway. Show the portrait board to your partner, and brag about yourself. Yes, we know, you're not supposed to brag on yourself. But in this instance, the goal is to understand and know yourself better, not to put somebody else down, so do your best. Point out your good qualities, and how you have arranged the board to show them. Listen to the boasts of your partner. If your partner leaves out or diminishes some of the qualities that you mentioned, point that out. Never allow any dissension during this exercise.

Say, "thank you" to your partner.

Take a week off, before the next assignment.

THREE QUALITIES ABOUT MY PARTNER THAT I ADMIRE	INSTANCES WHEN I RECOGNIZED THE QUALITY
1.	
2.	
3.	

THREE QUALITIES ABOUT MY PARTNER THAT I ADMIRE	INSTANCES WHEN I RECOGNIZED THE QUALITY
1.	
2.	
3.	

Evie and Sandra

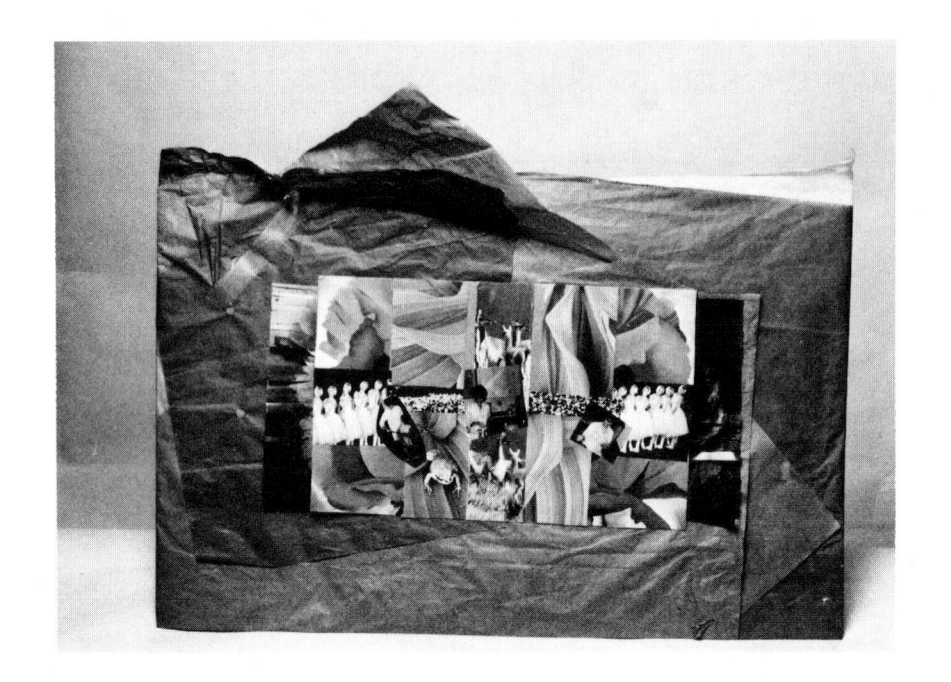

Evie: "This assignment had an impact on me, because intellectually I know the things that my partner said to me. She said (1) that I was good at making a confrontation seem valuable rather than brutal, (2) that I am a fine clinician, a master at my work, and (3) that I am able to articulate complex ideas. I "knew" all those things, but putting myself in a concrete picture owning it and putting it down and saying, "yes, this is who I am" went against all of that "tooting my own horn" business, and I felt a little grandiose. It's all right for somebody else to say, but it's a little bit inflated to say about myself. So it was difficult and I was surprised by that, surprised a lot."

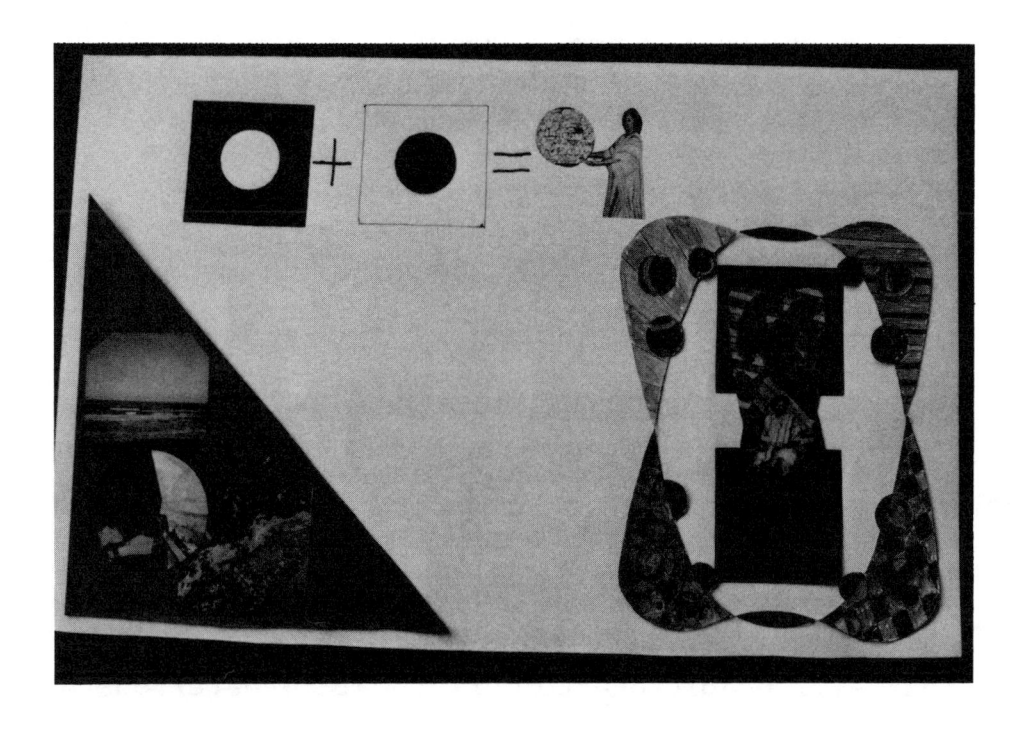

Sandra: "Blind spots. My partner said that the three things that she perceived about me are (1) I am a good problem solver, (2) I am comfortable with myself and (3) I know how to say hard things to people in a way that they feel they have been supported. And that's why I have this framework with all the doodads and bright colors, so that I can use the colors to distract people from knowing what is really going on. The picture at the top represents my problem solving and I do think that I do that well and sometimes very well when necessary. My triangle in the corner shows me being very comfortable at the beach which is where these pictures were taken when we were on retreat. I am the most comfortable with myself when I am at the beach and in this setting."

SECTION THREE: WHERE AM I NOW AND WHERE AM I GOING?

Assignment # 6: Visual Transitions

Brief Explanation

Change is very difficult. Often people have insight into needed changes, but lack the ability to actually make the change. Many psychotherapists have suggested implementing small changes in behavior that will enable one to work toward greater changes. The metaphorical change, created by you with the photographs and the art work, represents such an implementation.

One of the most innovative psychotherapists of our time, the late Milton Erickson, was a proponent of small changes. He often wrote that if a pattern can be changed in some small way, there is the possibility for further change. Many of the psychotherapy methods he developed were designed to encourage and facilitate small changes (Rossi, 1980).

Jean Houston writes, "To change the modality we must change the metaphor. In our research we have found the metaphors which provide for the personalizing of body parts and states can often give us the charged imagery that then creates those channels of communication for dialogue with our innate body image." (1982, p.12).

"Visual Transitions" provides a structure for you to create, through photographs and art work, your present state and also a more preferred state, indicating a new level of coping. The photographs and the art work are combined to reveal the relationship between these two states. Through movement and discussion with your partner, you will experience metaphorically the transition from your present state to the more preferred state. This metaphorical transition then paves the way for the more complicated and difficult changes that are desired in "real life."

Supplies Needed

1. Camera.
2. Film for two photographs each.
3. One sheet of poster board each.
4. Assorted art supplies, glue and scissors.

Assignment

Pose for two photographs, as you are now, and as you would like to be. Ask your partner for help in deciding on the poses. Get your partner to take the photographs then reciprocate.

Mount the two photographs on the poster board, representing

the relationship between the "now" and "then." At this point, don't worry about how you get from one to another. Using the art materials, relate the two somehow. If you can't figure out how to do it, just let your unconscious take over, and start playing around with the materials. You will find that the photos and art materials will fall into place without conscious effort on your part.

Processing

Look at your two poses on the poster board, and label each of them. Tell your partner what the labels are. Use labels with one or two words. Demonstrate, with your body, the first pose and ask your partner to imitate the pose. Both of you hold the pose and see how it feels. What associations does the pose evoke? Sometimes a pose will remind one of childhood experiences or unpleasant emotions. Repeat the modeling and imitation several times, and say the label out loud, both of you. Talk about how the pose makes you feel.

Model the second pose, and have your partner imitate it. Hold that pose and see how it feels. Talk about it. Repeat the modeling and imitation several times and say the label out loud.

Now move as fluidly as possible from the first pose to the second pose. Have your partner move with you. Repeat the movement several times until it is smooth and fluid. As you move, notice the different body sensations, and what bodily changes are necessary for making the transition from your present state to the more desired one. Experience the constriction of the first pose and the freedom of the second.

Help your partner with her processing, in the same manner. As she models and labels her poses and movements, imitate those and move along with her.

Talk about the art work and the experience of the movement. Explain your poster board to your partner. You may want to add to your board at this point. Many people feel the need to add another photograph to the two already there, sometimes to represent a middle point, or to depict the realization that the second pose was, itself, an interim point and further change is desired. The added photo is necessary to show the added change. Make any modifications you want. Discuss the modifications with your partner. Model, label and imitate any added poses.

One last thing. Discuss with your partner how you can now begin to make any desired changes in your life. Make no promises or vows, but simply explore possibilities. Listen to your partner as she discusses her beginnings of change.

Take a break for a few days. Give your new understanding and new learning time to become integrated into your personality.

Put the poster board someplace where you can see it every day.

<u>Evie and Sandra</u>

Evie and Sandra discuss their <u>visual transitions</u> work after the next assignment.

SECTION FOUR: WHAT IS IN THE WAY?

Assignment # 7:   Letting Go of Blocks

Brief Explanation

What are blocks? Blocks are whatever you do or say to yourself that interfere with doing whatever you want to do. For example, a block is saying to yourself that you are too old or too young, too tired or too lazy, too tall or too short, too dumb or too ignorant.

Do these sound familiar?

"I would go back to school, but I would be 36 years old by the time I graduate!"

"Who would want to go out with someone like me?"

"I would apply for that job but they've probably already hired somebody."

"I just don't have a head for math!"

"But I don't have any experience in that area!"

"What if she says no?"

"I just have too much going on right now to take on anything else."

"What if it rains?"

Blocks are one kind of self-talk that the psychiatrist Harry Stack Sullivan called Security Operations (1953). Security Operations are what we do to maintain the status quo, to keep from taking any chances on rejection or failure. Blocks can be summarized by the self-statement, "If I don't take a chance, then I won't get hurt." And they work. Not taking chances, not venturing to change, is safe.

We must assume, however, that because you are in this program you are wanting to change, to take a risk, to try for a better life. In this assignment, we will help you to recognize what blocks you are throwing up in front of yourself, and to help you deal with them. Sometimes blocks can be simply dissolved. Other times they can be skirted. Still others can be hurtled. Large blocks, barricades, must be either dismantled or circumvented.

Supplies Needed

1. Camera.
2. Film for one photograph each.
3. Art Work from Visual Transitions assignment.

4. One sheet of poster board.

5. Assorted art supplies, glue and scissors.

Assignment

Pick up your poster board work from the <u>visual transitions</u> assignment. Look at it and remind yourself about the change you portrayed in that assignment. Briefly describe the change to your partner, using the labels you assigned to the two poses.

Tell your partner three reasons why you want to change.

Now, tell your partner three reasons why you can't move from pose one to pose two. Use the statement, "I can't move from (label for pose 1) to (label for pose 2) because _____. Repeat the statement three times, giving a different reason each time.

Choose one of the reasons. Discuss with your partner how you could pose for a picture dealing with that reason, that block. Tell your partner what the block does for you, how it serves you. How would you symbolically portray the block? How would you symbolically deal with it? You might picture yourself skirting around it, hurtling it, dissolving it, blowing it up, or dismantling it. Very large blocks, barricades you might say, will have to be dealt with in dramatic ways. It might be possible to portray barricades in stages or parts, and deal with each part separately.

Let your partner take a picture of you dealing with the block. You will probably then want to use the other art materials to depict the block, or to add to the detail, on the <u>visual transitions</u> poster board. The end result will be a modification of the visual transitions work that will show not only the visual transition, but yourself dealing with whatever block is in the way of achieving that change, of making that transition. If you do not want to modify your visual transitions work, then show the block and yourself dealing with it on a separate sheet of poster board.

In a similar program several years ago, a man portrayed his visual transition as wanting to move from "apathy" to "getting things done." The label "apathy" was applied to a picture of himself bogged down in a swamp. The label "getting things done" was applied to a picture of himself striding confidently down a road. Later, he realized that he was blocking himself by trying to concentrate on unimportant details rather than what really needed to be done. For example, he would count paper clips, sharpen his pencil, worry about whether he had enough paper. The swamp was the morass of details that he used to avoid doing the more relevant parts of his job. He stayed in the swamp because it was safe. He was very good at counting paper clips and sharpening pencils. No possibility of failure there. Writing a report, however, and presenting it in a staff meeting, was risky. Symbolically, he portrayed the solution to the block by drawing in an elevated highway above the swamp, connecting to the "getting things done" road, with another picture of himself walking along that road, skirting the swamp of petty details. That road he labeled "competence and confidence." At the end of that exercise he remarked in wonder, "For years I have been wading through the swamp and there was a road there all the time!"

By now you know that these assignments apply to both you and your partner. Help your partner with his or her photographs and art work.

Processing

Describe your art work to your partner. Discuss, in particular, how you dealt with the block metaphorically. How did it feel? Show your partner by re-enacting the pose, how you handled the block. Have your partner enact the pose with you. Feel the power and competence that pose evokes.

Now, tell your partner three reasons why you <u>can</u> move from pose one to pose two of the <u>visual transition</u>. Use the statement, "I <u>can</u> move from (label for pose 1) to (label for pose 2) because _____. In the example above, the man stated, "I can move from apathy to getting things done because I am competent." "I can move from apathy to getting things done because I don't need to count paper clips, I have the resources I need." If you have problems thinking of three reasons, ask your partner for help. Remember your strengths, from the assignment on blind spots. Those strengths are not blind spots any more. You can see them clearly. Use them to overcome blocks.

Evie and Sandra

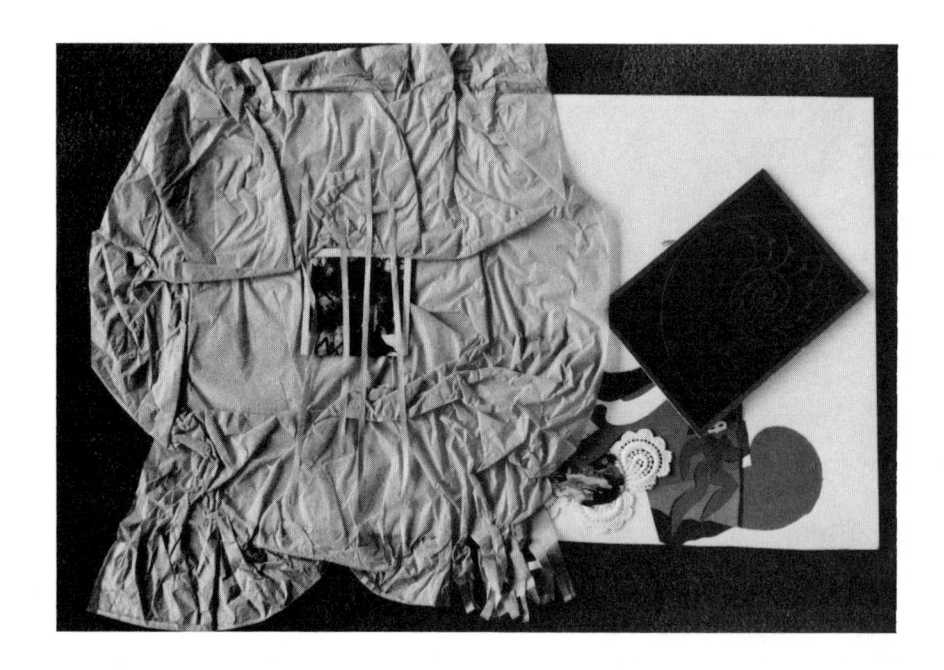

Evie: "This is a combined poster of the way I see myself now, the way I'd like to be and what it's going to take to get there. I started on the left with the way it is now with a sort of imprisonment in a set of fuzzy standards that I never quite measure up to. I've been catching a lot of that in trying to get a training institute into a regularized curriculum, moving from a creative way of doing psychodrama into a predictable curriculum that people can follow and depend on, one that won't change on them, one that keeps all their records straight, all of the "stuff" of administration. I'm always feeling caught up by the details. Even a small typo is cause for somebody to rub my nose in the fact that I am doing it "wrong." Somehow I am really sensitive to all of that right now. It's giving me a lot of trouble with my relationships. So that's where I am at the moment.

Where I would like to be is not quite such an open book, so it's inside a card. Although the card has easy access, it takes a little effort to open it up. It contains a much more relaxed pose, not standing back by the tree with a measuring rod, but seated on a rock, comfortable because I know I've done the best job I can do. It's not perfect, it'll never be perfect, and furthermore it doesn't have to be perfect. This is just where it is right now.

Assignment seven was to look at how to get there. I think the way to get there is to handle it with a much lighter touch, to play with it more, to laugh at it more, to not get into the game of having to defend myself. Take it to Mardi Gras. Feed the ducks. Do things that are not so serious all the time. It only serves to hook people's resentments about authority. I don't need that."

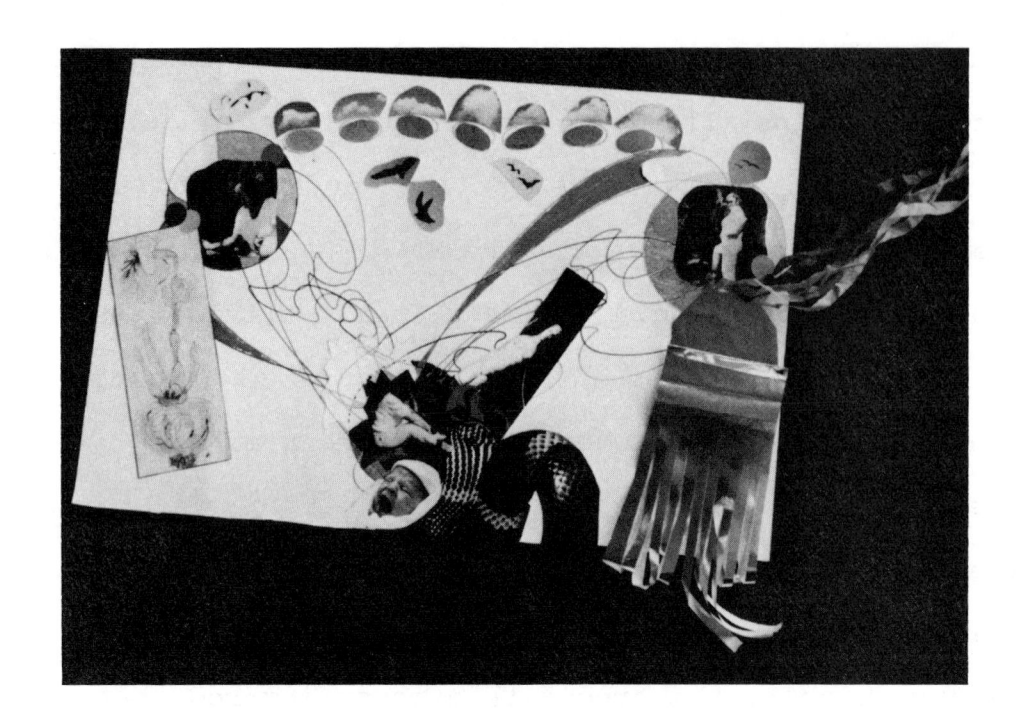

Sandra: "My first pose shows me questioning why I have to change my lifestyle in order to give myself a healthy body. This is an ongoing theme I am working on through this set of assignments I am doing. In this photo art therapy assignment, I want to be standing victorious in a healthy body, and I have a picture of that on the far right side.

The blocks that I have that keep me from doing this is the picture in the center and it shows me full of apathy and depression and drinking too much and eating too much. It's got a snake that's full of temptation for me to do all the things that I used to think were exciting, and it also shows a baby's crying face. Sometimes I feel like a baby, and I cry about the things that I don't want to do.

The way I can move from where I am to where I want to be is by doing it one step at a time, and I've shown that with the clouds.

To fly is the way to move and if I can somehow figure out a way to be with the birds and fly across and take it lightly and do it happily I think that is going to work for me. I can move from being unhealthy to healthy because I desire it. I want to be healthy so I can continue my work and I have the discipline to follow through with my program."

Assignment #8: Resolving Conflicts

Brief Explanation

By conflicts, we mean internal conflicts, not conflicts between people. Conflicts pull in different directions at the same time, and therefore use up energy that you could use to move in the direction of more satisfaction and fulfillment. As long as you are fighting yourself, it is difficult to make any movement at all.

In their simplest forms, there are three types of conflicts, approach-approach, avoidance-avoidance, and approach-avoidance. Approach-approach conflicts arise when you have two equally desirable goals, and you can't decide on which one because you want both an equal amount. Shall I have chocolate ice cream or strawberry? Which job offer shall I accept? The great thing about approach-approach conflicts is that you can't lose. Whichever decision you make, you win. You can only lose if you put off making the decision until neither alternative is still available. That happens sometimes, but rarely. Approach-approach conflicts are win-win situations.

Avoidance-avoidance conflicts are lose-lose situations, and usually arise because of external pressures. Many young men were confronted with an extreme avoidance-avoidance conflict during the Vietnam war when they tried to decide whether to register for the draft, and possibly be killed, or to flee to Canada, and become expatriates. Neither alternative was desirable. Your husband beats you, but the alternative is to leave him and go on welfare with no place to stay.

Avoidance-avoidance conflicts put you "between the devil and the deep blue sea." "Between a rock and a hard place." You're "damned if you do and damned if you don't." As you can see, we have plenty of sayings to describe avoidance-avoidance conflicts. One more--we have to "make the best of a bad situation." "Making the best" usually means that the two alternatives are not truly equal. One of the alternatives has fewer bad consequences than the other. It is good to gain as much information about possible consequences as can be gained.

Approach-avoidance conflicts give us a great deal of psychological trouble, in the form of anxiety. Approach-avoidance conflicts arise when one goal has both positive and negative consequences, and we both desire and fear the same outcome. You want to get married and you don't. You want to go to college and you don't. You want a child and you don't. As the approach-avoidant goal comes closer, you become increasingly agitated, indecisive, and upset. You may try to "handle" the conflict by postponing it. So you postpone your wedding date, postpone enrolling, postpone your pregnancy. Then, a few days or weeks later, you become agitated, indecisive, and upset all over again.

It is possible to maintain this cycle of anxiety, postponement, and further anxiety indefinitely, and people do.

Why can't people resolve their conflicts without undue anguish? For one thing, they may not be able to see the conflict clearly. For another, they may be exaggerating the probabilities of certain outcomes. Also, people sometimes set things up so that a particular undesirable outcome is practically guaranteed. People also keep conflicts alive so that they never have to experience the outcome, no matter what it is, even with approach-approach conflicts. It is safer to live with anxiety than with action. Safer, but not very satisfying.

How can this photo art therapy assignment help? It can help in four ways:
1. By providing a format for looking at all sides of a conflict.
2. By making the outcomes tangible and concrete.
3. By helping you see how you may be engaging in self-defeating strategies.
4. By encouraging a metaphorical resolution of the conflict.

Supplies Needed

1. Camera.

2. Film for three photographs each.
3. One sheet of poster board each.
4. Assorted art materials, glue and scissors.

Assignment

Consider the discussion about conflicts, above. Choose one conflict that you are involved with at present. We all have many conflicts, so the difficult part is not to think of one but to choose which one you want to address. Talk about your choice with your partner. In particular, in your discussion with your partner, try to get a clear idea of the two sides of the conflict. Decide, with the help of your partner, how you can portray both sides of the conflict with two photographs of yourself. At this point concentrate on how to depict the conflict, not on how to resolve it. Pose for the two sides and have your partner take the photographs. Reciprocate with your partner. Take her photographs.

Using the photographs and the art materials, depict the conflict clearly on the background of the poster board. Cut out the images if you wish, and add anything you want with the art supplies. <u>Do not glue anything down yet</u>.

Processing

As you did during the <u>visual transitions</u> assignment, reenact for your partner the poses you used to portray both sides of the conflict. Get your body into one of the poses, and think of a one-word label for the pose. As you maintain the pose, say the label out loud. Ask your partner to assume the same pose and say the word with you. Now repeat that with the other side of the conflict. Move back and forth between the two poses, paying attention to the body tensions and feelings that represent both sides of the conflict. Attend to any similarities between the two poses.

Pay close attention to your body sensations, and now change each pose slightly in the direction of the other one. Demonstrate those two poses, and have your partner mirror your movements. Change the two poses slightly again, still in the direction of each other. You and your partner move through these two new poses. Each time you change poses to lessen the distance between the two sides, think up new labels, and say the labels out loud. Keep changing the poses toward a middle ground, and changing the labels that describe the poses, until you reach a single pose that is halfway between the two original sides of the conflict. Label that halfway point with a word or phrase. Have your partner take your picture in that pose. Symbolically, that new pose represents a resolution of the conflict.

Describe your art work to your partner. Describe your pictorial conflict as completely as you can. Ask your partner if he has seen anything you have overlooked. Thinking only of the art materials, how might the metaphorical conflict be changed? What would happen if you changed shapes, or colors, or the composition of the piece? Experiment with it. Change it. Now add your third picture to the art work wherever it fits best. Describe your new composition to your partner. When you are satisfied with it, glue everything down permanently.

Reciprocate. Listen to your partner's description, watch your partner's poses, mirror them. Help him as he helped you.

Display your art work where you will see it frequently. Wait a week before you begin the next assignment.

Evie and Sandra

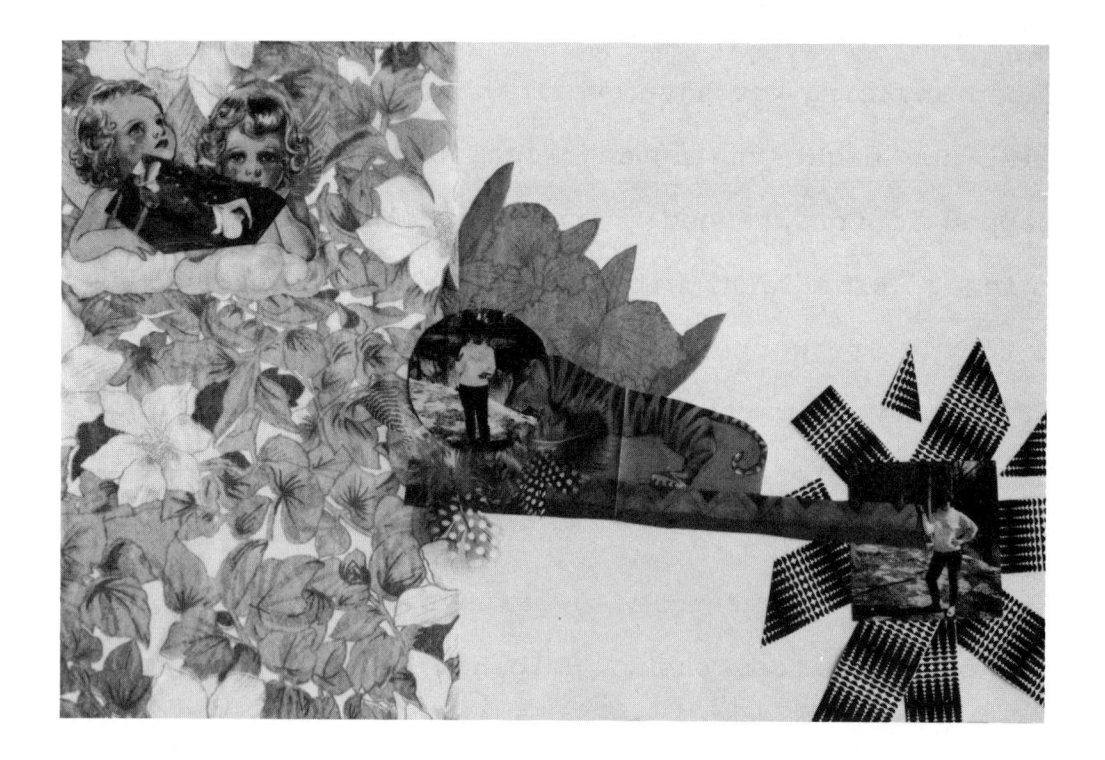

Evie: "Conflicts. My poster depicts on the left a really passive approach to the conflict I am having right now with the training group. Part of me wants to lie down and go to sleep and hope that it will solve itself by magic. It'll just go away. People will wake up and see the folly of their own ways without my having to do anything at all about it. That's the way it ought to be, part of me says.

The other part of me, on the far right, can really get into my activist stance and take a sort of New York-behind-the-barricade-in-the-sixties 'up yours' attitude and say, 'You guys are going to shape up or else you're not going to get any kind of certification ever out of this institute or out of me.'

Surely, somewhere, there is a medium space between these two.

I'm not sure I have discovered it yet, but there is a way to take a reasonable stance, one that says, 'This is simply the way it is.' A stance that is very firm, but not delivered with a sledge hammer, simply delivered. That's what I am working toward. Maybe with that picture in mind I will do a little bit better, because neither end of this spectrum is working very well for me."

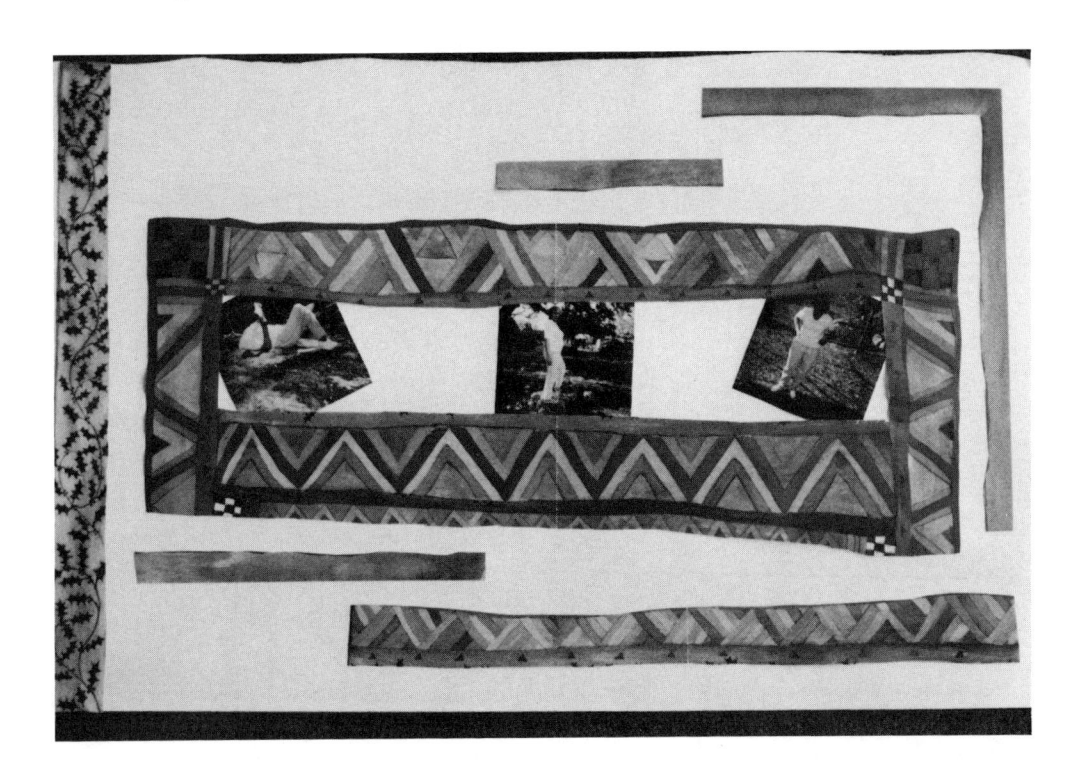

Sandra: "This is another poster about my health issue. My internal conflict about my health has avoidance on the left side and anger on the right side. As I do this poster I begin to see how self-defeating either one of these stances can be. They don't really work.

My metaphorical solution is to take one step at a time to resolution. The picture of the ivy on the left is to remind me that this can be a growth situation. I can really use this problem that I have to get to a new place, to a new understanding of myself and my body. I have all the bright colored framework around it because I am trying to reframe it in a way that will work."

SECTION FIVE: WHO ARE WE?

Assignment # 9:   Defining Our Partnership

Brief Explanation

You and your partner have been through quite an experience these past several weeks. Perhaps you knew each other only casually before beginning these assignments. If so, you now know each other very well. If you knew each other intimately before beginning the program, we think you will agree that you know each other much more intimately by now. You have listened, empathized, shared, understood. Because of the shared intensity of the program up to this point, and your changing relationship because of that intensity, it is time to redefine your partnership. It is time to ask, "Who are we?"

In this assignment, instead of helping each other make decisions, you will make joint decisions. The joint decision process will, in itself, help you to define your relationship more clearly.

Supplies Needed

1. Camera.
2. Film for at least two photographs.

3. One sheet of poster board.

4. Assorted art supplies, glue and scissors.

5. Art work from Assignment # 2.

Assignment

First, go back and review the assignment on "Who am I in relation to other people?" In particular, review the part concerning your relationship to people of the same gender as your partner. Both of you, get out your art work from that assignment and briefly describe it to each other. Your basic stance toward other people will form the background for your relationship with your partner.

Together, discuss how you can show your relationship with at least two photographs. Your initial impulse may be to pose together. We suggest that it will be more enlightening if you don't. Rather than posing together, you can pose separately and join the two photos later in whatever way you can agree upon. Your discussion and decision about how to join the photographs will be an important step in defining your relationship. Furthermore, by taking individual pictures you preserve the important fact that you two, in addition to being partners, are individuals and will remain so.

Together, place the photographs on the poster board,

symbolically showing your relationship. You may need more than two photographs. Take as many as you need. Use any other art materials you need to augment the photographs on the background. Before adding anything, make sure that you and your partner agree to the addition.

Even something as seemingly simple as choice of color or placement may be highly meaningful to your partner. A participant in this assignment related to us, "...then a very interesting thing happened. No sooner had I put my picture there than (my partner) immediately started painting around it and closed me off completely. I felt suffocated and alone and rejected in that corner. It was very interesting that I had been very comfortable in that place until I allowed someone else to make me miserable."

Keep at it until you both are satisfied that the work is complete. Explain your reasons and discuss each addition and change as you make it. When you are finished, glue everything down.

Processing

If you have truly worked together on the assignment up to this point, there will be little processing necessary. However, now is the time to bring up any unfinished business from the assignment. If you merely pretended to agree, but privately resent a color, form, or placement, now is the time to bring it up. Talk it out before beginning the next assignment.

<u>Evie and Sandra</u>

Evie and Sandra discuss their work from assignment # 9 after the next assignment.

SECTION SIX: WHERE ARE WE NOW AND WHERE ARE WE GOING?

Assignment # 10: Visual Transitions As Partners

Brief Explanation

This assignment parallels Assignment # 6, but this time as partners rather than as individuals. The first part of your visual transition as partners assignment is already finished. Assignment # 9 asked you to define your relationship. By definition, that is your relationship as it is now. Now, take that assignment a step further and explore your relationship as you imagine or hope it will be in the future.

Probably you and your partner have both similar and different fantasies about where your relationship is headed. A clear understanding about those differences and some agreement about similarities would be helpful in avoiding future clashes and disappointments.

Supplies Needed

1. Camera.
2. Film for at least two photographs.
3. One sheet of poster board.
4. Assorted art supplies, glue and scissors.

5. Art work from assignment # 9.

Assignment

You will need your art work from the previous assignment. Get that out now, and review it. That art work depicts your "Who are we now?" part of the assignment. You will add the "Where are we going?" part by creating a second poster board to go with the first.

As you did with the previous assignment, discuss with your partner how you can create a poster board that will depict your ideal relationship sometime in the future. When you have an understanding and agreement as to how that future relationship can be depicted using photographs of the two of you, pose for those photographs and take each other's picture. Discuss and agree on the placement of the photographs on the blank piece of poster board. Use at least two photographs, and more if you wish.

Using the other art materials, add whatever needs to be added to the poster board. Remember to discuss and agree before adding anything.

Processing

Place the two completed poster boards next to each other, the one from assignment # 9 and the one just finished. Now, as you did with the individual <u>visual transition</u> assignment, reposition your bodies in the same relationship as the photographs in the "Who are We?" poster. Agree on a label for the pose. Now pose as in the "Where are we going?" poster and agree on that label. Say the labels out loud as you assume the poses. Assume the first pose again and move from the first to the second, saying the two labels as you move from one to the other. Pay particular attention to your physical relationship as you move from one set of poses to the other. Talk about it.

If necessary, take additional photographs and modify the poster boards. Discuss and agree on everything before gluing down permanently or adding ink or paint.

Shake hands.

Take a break for a week.

Evie and Sandra

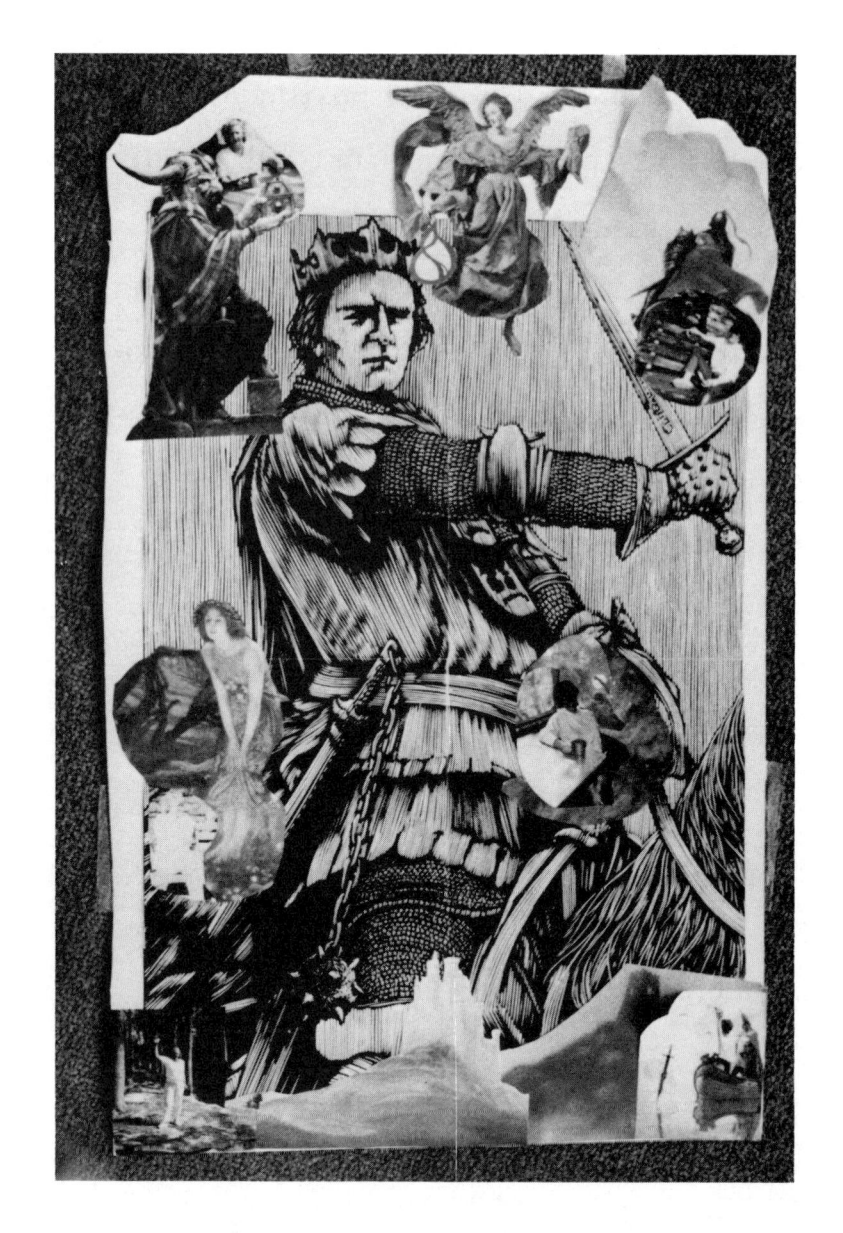

Evie: " Assignment 9 and 10, 'Who we are as partners.' This one was wonderful to do together, really fun and creative which I think says a lot about our partnership. We chose mythological figures because we had so much fun with this whole adventure. It feels like we are both in our 'adventuring' stance, our 'warrior' cycle, having decided what it is we wanted to do and having found the courage to stick with it and do it. Put it into action. It's been great fun."

Sandra: "Our picture shows us drinking coffee, talking, planning, sharing and helping each other as we go forth to do battle in the business world. We are both very aware of our guardian angel that has been with us from the beginning. she floats over the top of everything we do and holds the Innerstages logo safely and carefully in her hand."

Evie: "We are aware of both 'magical' qualities that have been involved, and also what it's taken on our own parts to bring this into fruition. At the bottom is a picture of how we want it to be--free to go in different directions because we have done our homework: We have drunk enough coffee together; we have sat on enough benches together; we know from the inside out that this thing is on a very firm footing and so either one of us can get in a boat and sail away or walk down a path that's separate and not put in jeopardy this venture we've undertaken together. Our partnership won't be jeopardized by it."

Sandra: "As we venture out to gather more information and have more experiences, we know we have Innerstages to come back to and share that richness with each other so that we can both grow. This has been an incredible experience, not only to do this photo art therapy session together, but to help us highlight and understand how important our relationship is as friends, as colleagues, and as business partners. I love the metaphor of the warriors and the going forth to do battle, and castles in the background that show us that we do have a home and it will be there waiting for us."

<u>Evie:</u> "It's a many, many faceted jewel that we hold up and it is difficult to keep all of the different roles separate. They are never entirely separate and so we work through all of this richness, spending a lot of time at it so that one of the facets doesn't get messed up, thereby messing up all of them. The tapestry is complex."

SECTION SEVEN: WHERE HAVE I BEEN THESE PAST FEW WEEKS?

Assignment # 11: Review And Summary

Brief Explanation

It is hardly necessary to justify a review and summary. In any program of several weeks duration, participants will have forgotten some of the experiences, there will be some lingering questions or doubts, and there will be a lack of closure.

Now is your chance to summarize all of the experiences of the past few weeks. It is also your chance to express anything to your partner that you have been suppressing or censoring. Finally, this assignment will give you a sense of completion, of closure.

Supplies Needed

1. All art work from previous assignments.
2. Camera.
3. Film for at least one photograph each.
4. One sheet of poster board each.
5. Assorted art supplies, glue and scissors.

Assignment

You and your partner arrange all of your art work around the room so that you can view it all at once. Arrange it in order of the assignments. If you need more space, find it. You can go outdoors, or to a classroom somewhere, or a studio.

Begin with assignment #1 and both you and your partner discuss and reminisce about the assignment. Try to remember how you felt about it at the time you did it, and how you feel about it now. Continue with assignment #2 and so on until you discuss all of the pieces of work.

Pose for a photograph (or more than one, if you wish) that symbolizes your journey of the past few weeks. Have your partner take the photograph, then help her with her poses and photographs. Mount the photograph or photographs on a sheet of poster board and represent your summary of the entire program experience by augmenting the photographs with the art materials. Let your partner help you decide on the poses. Help her.

Processing

Show and describe your poster board to your partner. Listen to her description of her poster. Talk about how the program has influenced you, and what you got out of it. Talk about the things that bothered you. Talk with your partner how you might implement some of the learning you have done these past few weeks, to better your life. <u>Make no promises.</u> Simply explore possibilities.

Thank your partner for all of the help and understanding.

<u>Evie and Sandra</u>

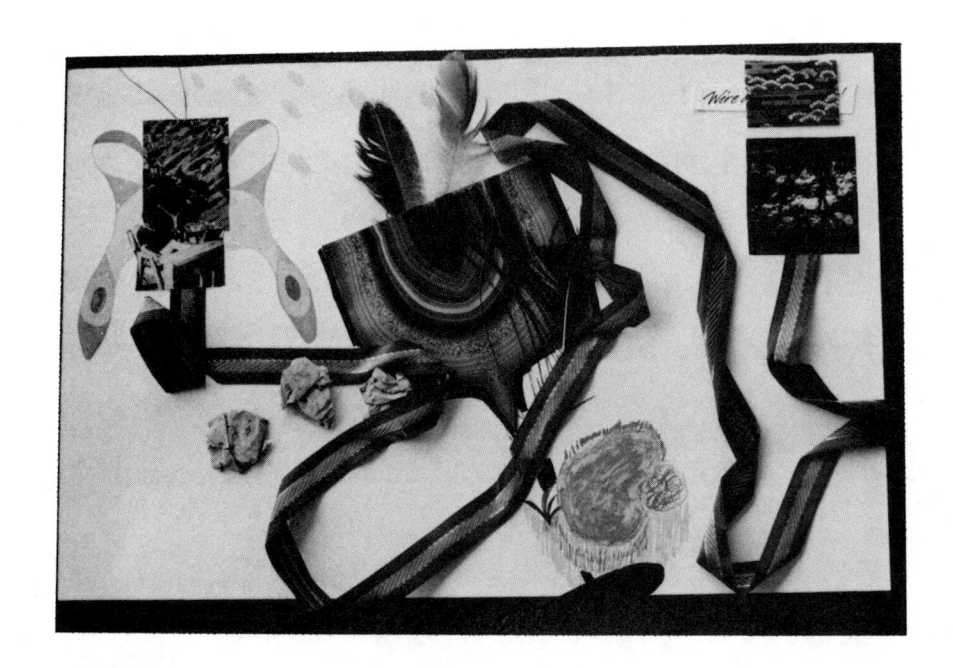

<u>Evie:</u> "The journey, where it started and where it's gone and where we are now. We started this photo art therapy project at the beginning of our opening the doors of the Institute, so I went back to all of the daydreaming, fantasizing, that we did before we started our process here. We did it in a variety of settings over a long time, but a lot of dreaming went into this.   Then the road along the way was not a straight and narrow path by any means. It went around rocks and over hills and through some celebrations

and through some swamp land and finally launched us into the river. I feel like we are not at the beginning stages any more, but that we are in process. The good Lord only knows where it's all going but it feels like we are in the river.

At the very, very top is a little message, 'We are a winning team.' We've had to learn through a very difficult process with friends and colleagues that the winning team can't hang out in public all the time. It needs to be a private awareness. between us. That's been a difficult thing to learn, but valuable.

So somehow this photo art therapy project has been with us along all of these different steps. It's been used to work out internal conflicts. It's been used to work out and clarify our relationship and at the end of this we are launched!"

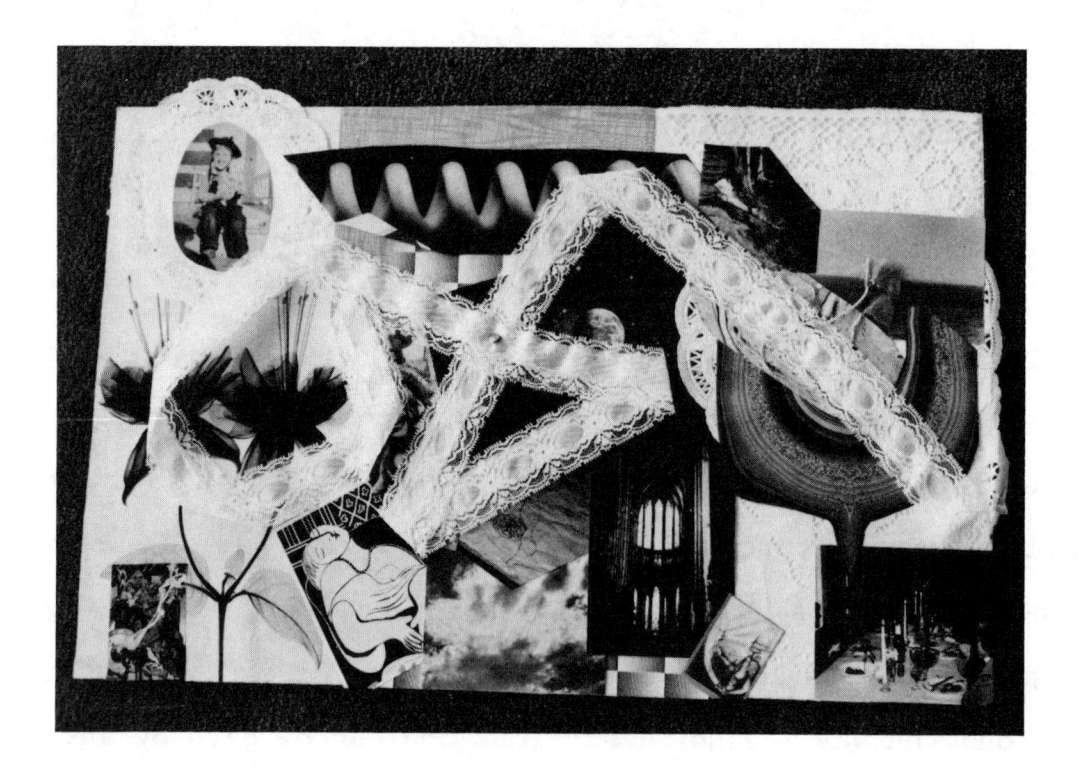

Sandra: "I found that my life journey has been very similar

to the journey I have made during this photo art therapy session. I have a picture at the upper left hand corner of myself when I was four or five years old and my name was Sissy. I am sitting on the steps waiting to start an adventure, excited, happy and ready to go. That Sissy is connected across the top of the page to myself as I am today, sitting on a slide, sliding down into a river. This river called Innerstages, our Company, is carrying me on a voyage that is exciting and full of contentment and joy. I feel like I am floating down a river doing what I ought to be doing effortlessly, being held safely by some sort of natural urn as I have portrayed in this picture. The voyage has a celebration of life in the picture in the bottom right hand side. The journey from Sissy to Sandra at Innerstages has covered a lot of territory. The pictures show myself as a potter, as a mother, and when I was blue skying my way across the world. It shows the body work I've done, my interest in science and quantum physics, and my transformational experience in a cathedral in Cologne that changed my life and sent me in the direction of Innerstages.

This real journey has been full of joy, beauty, excitement and sometimes pain and frustration. The photo art therapy journey has been sometimes full of pain and frustration as well but I see it has been worth it. This summary picture tells me that the journey was good and that the mistakes I made along the way are minor and not nearly as important as the victories."

REFERENCES

Feininger, A. (1956). <u>The anatomy of nature.</u> New York: Dover Publications, Inc.

Feininger, A. (1977). <u>Nature close up: A fantastic journey unto reality.</u> New York: Dover Publications, Inc.

Feininger, A. (1983). <u>Nature and art: A photographic exploration.</u> New York: Dover Publications, Inc.

Feininger, A. (1986). <u>In a grain of sand: Exploring design by nature.</u> San Francisco: Sierra Club Books.

Hall, J. (1990). Presentation at conference on C. G. Jung, University of Houston-Clear Lake, Houston, Texas.

Houston, J. (1982). <u>The possible human.</u> Los Angeles: J. P. Tarcher.

Jung, C. G. (1968). <u>The archetypes and the collective unconscious.</u> Vol. 9, Part 1, of the <u>Collected works of C. G. Jung.</u> Princeton: Princeton University Press.

McNiff, S. (1987). Pantheon of creative arts therapies: An integrative image of the profession. <u>Journal of Integrative</u>

and Eclectic Therapy. 6(3), 259-281.

Rossi, E. L. (Ed.) (1980). *The collected papers of Milton H. Erickson on hypnosis, Vols. I-IV.* New York: Irvington Publishers, Inc.

Schutz, W. C. (1958). *FIRO: A three-dimensional theory of interpersonal behavior.* New York: Holt, Rinehart and Co., Inc.

Sullivan, H. S. (1953). *The interpersonal theory of psychiatry.* (H. S. Perry and M. L. Gawel, Eds.). New York: Norton.

Wadeson, H. (1980). *Art psychotherapy.* New York: Wiley.

SOME FURTHER READING

Dalley, T., Case, C., Schaverien, J., Weir, F., Halliday, D., Hall, P. N., and Waller, D. (1987). *Images of art therapy: New developments in theory and practice.* London: Tavistock.

Feder, E. and Feder, B. (1981) *The expressive arts therapies.* Englewood Cliffs, NJ: Prentice Hall.

Fleshman, B. and Fryrear, J. L. (1981) *The arts in therapy.* Chicago, IL: Nelson-Hall.

Fryrear, J. L. and Corbit, I. E. (1992) *Photo art therapy: A Jungian perspective.* Springfield, IL: Charles C Thomas.

Hattersley, R. (1971) *Discover yourself through photography.* New York: Morgan and Morgan.

Krauss, D. and Fryrear, J. L. (1983) *Phototherapy in mental health.* Springfield, IL: Charles C Thomas.

Landgarten, H. (1981) *Clinical art therapy: A comprehensive guide.* New York: Brunner/Mazel.

Liebmann, M. (1986) <u>Art therapy for groups: A handbook of themes, games and exercises.</u> London: Croom Helm. Cambridge, MA: Brookline Books.

McNiff, S. (1981) <u>The arts and psychotherapy.</u> Springfield, IL: Charles C Thomas.

McNiff, S. (1988) <u>Fundamentals of art therapy.</u> Springfield, IL: Charles C Thomas.

Naumberg, M. (1950) <u>An introduction to art therapy.</u> New York: Teachers College Press.

Nucho, A. (1987) <u>The psychocybernetic model of art therapy</u>. Springfield, IL: Charles C Thomas.

Rhyne, J. (1973) <u>The gestalt art experience.</u> Monterey, CA: Brooks/Cole.

Robbins, A. and Sibley, L. (1973) <u>Creative art therapy.</u> New York: Brunner/Mazel.

Robbins, A. (1987). <u>The artist as therapist.</u> New York: Human Sciences Press, Inc.

Rubin, J. (1984) *The art of art therapy.* New York: Brunner/Mazel.

Rubin, J. (1987). *Approaches to art therapy: Theory and technique.* New York: Brunner/Mazel.

Wadeson, H. (1980) *Art psychotherapy.* New York: Wiley.

Wadeson, H. (1987) *The dynamics of art psychotherapy.* New York: Wiley.

Wadeson, H., Durkin, J. and Perach, D., Eds. (1989) *Advances in art therapy.* New York: Wiley.

ABOUT THE AUTHORS

Jerry L. Fryrear, Ph.D., A.T.R., is a clinical psychologist and art therapist. He is professor of psychology at the University of Houston-Clear Lake and has a private practice in psychology and art therapy. Dr. Fryrear has published four books and numerous chapters and articles on the expressive arts in therapy. He is on the editorial board of <u>The Arts in Psychotherapy.</u>

Irene E. Corbit, Ph.D., A.T.R., LPC is an art therapist in private practice in Houston. She conducts workshops on the expressive arts in therapy, in addition to her work with private clients. She is coordinator of the School of The Expressive Arts at the C. G. Jung Educational Center in Houston. Dr. Corbit is on the editorial board of <u>The Arts in Psychotherapy</u> and is an adjunct instructor at the University of Houston-Clear Lake. Dr. Corbit and Dr. Jerry L. Fryrear have coauthored <u>Photo Art Therapy: A Jungian Perspective</u>, published in Summer, 1992.

Sandra Mason Taylor, M.A., LPC, LCDC, is a psychotherapist and Founder and President of Innerstages, Psychodrama Applications, Inc. She provides psychodrama therapy services to local psychiatric hospitals, out-patient clinics and medical practices. Ms. Taylor is licensed both as a Professional Counselor and a Chemical Dependency Counselor in the state of Texas.